hiking from here to

WOW

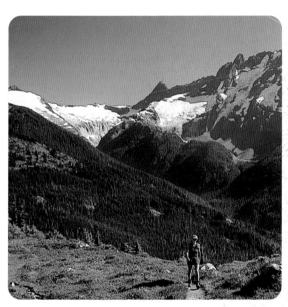

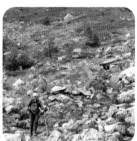

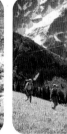

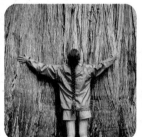

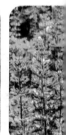

WOW GUIDES

NORTH
CASCADES

Kathy & Craig Copeland

WILDERNESS PRESS

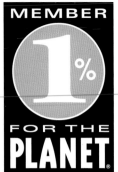

MEMBER 1% FOR THE PLANET

Businesses donating
1% of their sales to the
natural environment
www.onepercentfortheplanet.org
The authors are members.

Hiking from here to WOW: North Cascades

1st EDITION, May 2007

Copyright © 2007 by Craig and Kathy Copeland

All photos and original maps by the authors

Book and map production by Angela Lockerbie
(lockerbie@shaw.ca)

Cover and interior design by Matthew Clark
(www.subplot.com)

ISBN: 978-0-89997-444-6
UPC: 7-19609-97444-4

Manufactured in China

Published by: **Wilderness Press
1200 5th Street
Berkeley, CA 94710
(800) 443-7227; FAX (510) 558-1696
info@wildernesspress.com
www.wildernesspress.com**
Visit our website for a complete listing of our titles
and for ordering information.

Authors of opinionated guidebooks always welcome readers' comments.
Write them at nomads@hikingcamping.com

Cover photo: Mt. Baker, from Skyline Divide (Trip 6)

Back cover photos: Challenger Glacier, from Whatcom Pass (Trip 42); Tiger lily,
Green Mtn (Trip 34); Lake Chelan (Trip 50)

Title page photos: (large one) Mt. Shuksan, from Yellow Aster Butte trail (Trip 9);
(top middle) Yellow Aster basin; (bottom middle) cedar along North Fork Sauk River
(Trip 46); (top right) Liberty Cap (Trip 47); (bottom right) lupine on Heather trail (Trip 1)

YOUR SAFETY IS YOUR RESPONSIBILITY

Hiking and camping in the wilderness can be dangerous. Experience and preparation reduce risk, but will never eliminate it. The unique details of your specific situation
and the decisions you make at that time will determine the outcome. Always check the
weather forecast and current trail conditions before setting out. This book is not a sub-
stitute for common sense or sound judgment. If you doubt your ability to negotiate
mountain terrain, respond to wild animals, or handle sudden, extreme weather changes,
hike only in a group led by a competent guide. The authors and the publisher disclaim
liability for any loss or injury incurred by anyone using information in this book.

CONTENTS

Shoulder-Season Trips 10 / Maps 10 / Carry a Compass 11 / Physical Capability 12 / Leave Your Itinerary 12 / Wilderness Ethics 12 / Hiking With Your Dog 15 / Who's in Charge Around Here? 16 / Backcountry Permits 17 / Northwest Forest Pass 18 / Volunteer Trail Maintenance 19 / Cascadian Climate 20 / Scourge of the Cascades 21 / Battling Brush 22 / Cougars 22 / Bears 23 / Lightning 25 / Hypothermia 26

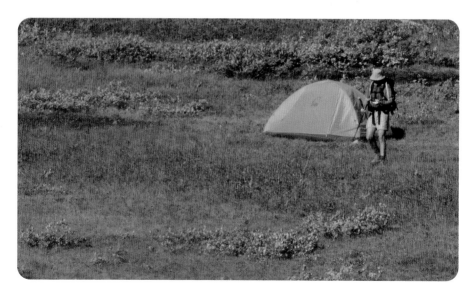

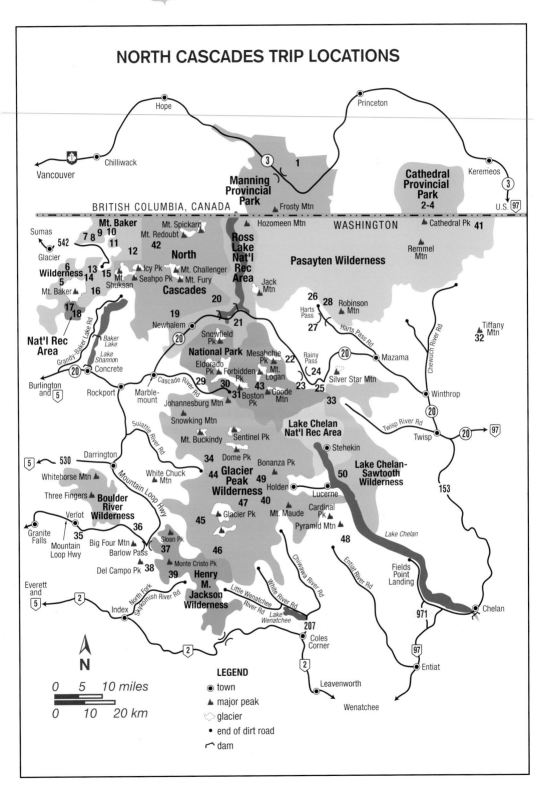

NORTH CASCADES TRIP LOCATIONS

Hope

Princeton

Chilliwack

Vancouver

Keremeos

Cathedral Provincial Park 2-4

Manning Provincial Park

1

BRITISH COLUMBIA, CANADA

Frosty Mtn

Sumas

542

Glacier

Mt. Baker
7 8 9 10
11

Mt. Spickard
Mt. Redoubt

12

42

Hozomeen Mtn

WASHINGTON

Cathedral Pk 41

Ross Lake Nat'l Rec Area

North

Remmel Mtn

6
Wilderness
5

13
14 15

16

Icy Pk Mt. Challenger
Seahpo Pk Mt. Fury

Pasayten Wilderness

Mt. Baker

Mt. Shuksan

Cascades

Jack Mtn

26   28 Robinson Mtn

Tiffany Mtn

17
18

Nat'l Rec Area

19

20

Harts Pass

27

32

Newhalem

Baker Lake

Lake Shannon

20

21

Snowfield Pk

Harts Pass Rd

Mazama

20

Burlington and 5

Concrete

Rockport

Marblemount

Cascade River Rd

National Park

Eldorado Pk Forbidden Pk

29   30

31 Boston Pk

43 Goode Mtn

Johannesburg Mtn

Mesahchie Pk 22

Mt. Logan

23   25

24

Rainy Pass

20

Silver Star Mtn

Winthrop

20

Twisp River Rd

33

Snowking Mtn

Mt. Buckindy

Sentinel Pk

Dome Pk

Lake Chelan Nat'l Rec Area

Stehekin

Twisp

20   97

Darrington

530

White Chuck Mtn

34

Bonanza Pk

Glacier Peak Wilderness

44

49

Holden

50

Lake Chelan-Sawtooth Wilderness

153

Whitehorse Mtn

Three Fingers **Boulder River Wilderness**

Verlot

35

36

Big Four Mtn

Barlow Pass

47   40

45

Sloan Pk

37

46

Lucerne

Cardinal Pk

Mt. Maude

Pyramid Mtn

48

Lake Chelan

Granite Falls

Mountain Loop Hwy

Del Campo Pk 38

39

Monte Cristo Pk

Henry M. Jackson Wilderness

Fields Point Landing

Chelan

Everett and 5

2

Index

North Fork Skykomish River Rd

Little Wenatchee River Rd

White River Rd

Chiwawa River Rd

Entiat River Rd

971

Lake Wenatchee

207

Coles Corner

97

Entiat

2

Leavenworth

Wenatchee

Suiattle River Rd

Mountain Loop Hwy

Glacier Pk

N

0   5   10 miles

0   10   20 km

LEGEND

town

major peak

glacier

end of dirt road

dam

50 TRAILS TO THE WONDER OF WILDERNESS

trip number / trip name / page number

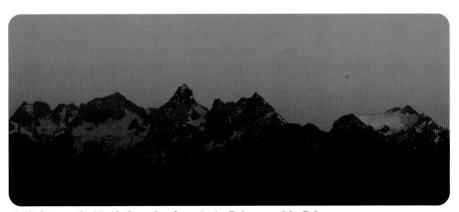

Twilight over the North Cascades, from Artist Point near Mt. Baker

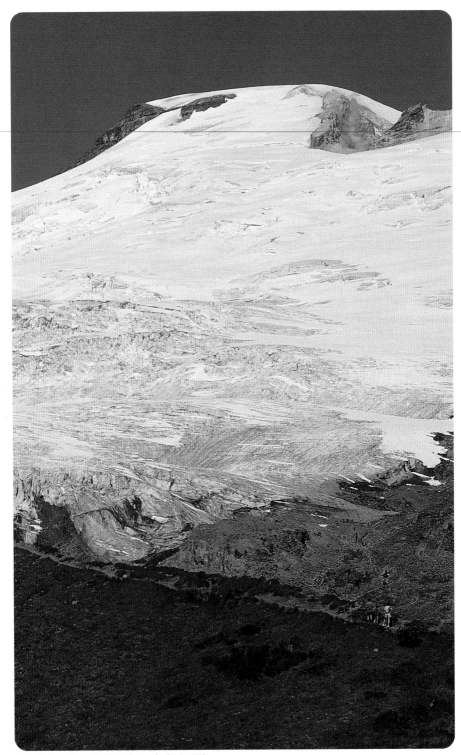

Mt. Baker, from Railroad Grade (Trip 17)

FROM HERE TO WOW

A disappointing trip leaves a psychic dent. Sometimes it can't be helped. But often it can, by knowing where to go instead of guessing.

Too many hikers toil up scenically deprived trails to lackluster destinations when they could be savoring one of North America's consummate mountain panoramas. That's been our motivation: to save you from wasting your precious time.

Even in this glorious mountain kingdom, not all scenery is created equal. Some places are simply more striking, more intriguing, more inspiring than others. Now you can be certain you're choosing the most rewarding trail for your weekend or vacation.

This isn't a catalog of every trail in the range. We wrote one a decade ago. Titled *Don't Waste Your Time in the North Cascades*, it detailed 110 trips. It's no longer available. Its offspring is the book you now hold in your hands.

A more focused volume covering only the premier trails is, we've discovered, a preferable resource for the majority of North Cascades hikers. So here you go: the 50 trails most likely to make you say "Wow!"

No okay trails. Not even any pretty good trails. And certainly no trudgemills. Just the dayhikes and backpack trips that will get you from here to WOW—the wonder of wilderness—as swiftly as possible. Plus our boot-tested opinions: why we recommend each trail, what to expect, how to enjoy the optimal experience.

Our assessments are based on widely shared, common-sense criteria. To help you understand our commentary, here are our preferences:

- A hike isn't emotionally satisfying solely because of the destination. We want to be wowed along the way by stately trees, profuse wildflowers, plunging gorges, rocky escarpments. Watching a stream charge on its journey is rapturous. Trails carved into rugged mountainsides are enthralling. Solitude is a sustaining necessity of life. Observing wild creatures is a primal joy. The closer we get to gleaming glaciers and piercing peaks, the more ecstatic we feel. High, airy, eye-stretching, soul-expanding perches thrill us most of all.
- Spending an entire, sunny, summer day below treeline doesn't appeal to us. Plodding for hours through disenchanted forest (scrawny, scrubby) is depressing. We soon lose interest in rubble-pile mountains devoid of sharp definition or sheer walls. When the scenery is monotonous and the trail cantankerous, it's trudgery. Although we'll push ourselves far and high for a grand sight, we're disappointed by an unengaging approach.

This is the guidebook we wish we had when we first drove Highway 20 through North Cascades National Park and peered up at 4000 vertical feet of forest. It was daunting. Views from the highway, near Colonial Creek for example, only hinted at possibilities. Where were all the peaks? The glaciers? The meadows? The alpine vistas?

We've long since learned the North Cascades is a world of wonders for hikers of all levels. Mountain magic is here in staggering abundance, if you know where to look. So keep reading.

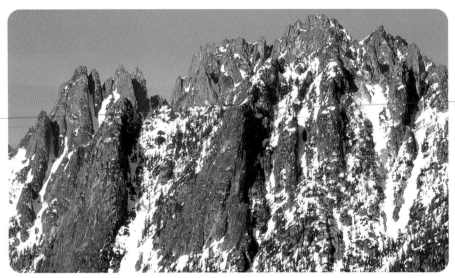

Early Winters Spires, from Washington Pass

We hope our suggestions compel you to get outdoors more often and stay out longer. Do it to cultivate your wild self. It will give you perspective. Do it because the backcountry teaches simplicity and self-reliance, qualities that make life more fulfilling. Do it to remind yourself why wilderness needs and deserves your protection. A bolder conservation ethic develops naturally in the mountains. And do it to escape the cacophony that muffles the quiet, pure voice within.

THE AMERICAN ALPS

According to the Bigfoot Field Researchers Organization (www.bfro.net), the state with the greatest number of credible Sasquatch sightings—more than 400 at last count—is Washington.

Maybe the elusive big guy is real. Maybe he's a hoax. One thing's for sure. No place else in the continental U.S. has such a high concentration of wild country. Sasquatch habitat, if you will, but definitely hiker habitat.

And at the heart of wild Washington are the North Cascades— enclave of spiky summits, colossal glaciers, psychedelic meadows, cathedral forests.

It's a shaggy, feral, volcano-studded range, with an atmosphere so prelapsarian it's no wonder people keep staggering out of the woods claiming to have seen monstrous creatures.

The name "North Cascades" refers to the abundance of sky-born waters cascading down these mountains. Myriad trickles, streams, creeks, rivers and falls nourish jungle-like biodiversity.

"The American Alps" is what President Lyndon Johnson called the range in his October 1968 Congressional address endorsing the creation of North Cascades National Park. The nickname stuck.

People fond of other U.S. mountains—the Sierra, the Rockies—occasionally try to usurp the adage. But anyone who's actually hiked throughout the American West knows better.

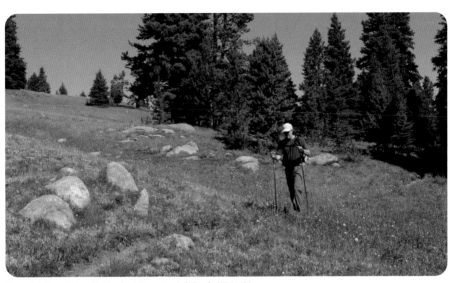

Scout Mountain, Cathedral Provincial Park (Trip 2)

The staff of Outward Bound, for example. In their North Cascades mountaineering course description, they invite you to "the American Alps," where you'll climb "open cliff faces" and explore "deep, glacially carved valleys," both of which are "characteristic of the European alpine environment."

But comparing the North Cascades with the Swiss Alps suggests only that the American version has a similar, equally impressive appearance. In other respects, anyone trying to fathom the range before they've hiked it should think Alaska.

In the U.S., only Alaska has more glacial ice than the North Cascades. And Mt. Baker's complex glaciation, which feeds three major river systems, is comparable to that of Alaskan peaks.

Mt. Shuksan, shouldering not just one glacier but four, and ice-laden Glacier Peak also do convincing impersonations of Alaskan mountains.

The North Cascades are also more Alaskan than European in terms of how remote they feel. Only one road, Hwy 20, traverses the range, and it's closed every winter due to heavy snows and avalanches.

Neither Europe nor Alaska, however, can claim the arboreal grandeur you'll witness in the North Cascades. Douglas firs, ponderosa pines, hemlocks, red cedars, and spruce grow so tall and girthy here, they inspire awe and reverence in all who pass.

Outside Washington state, the only place on earth whose mountains are truly akin to the North Cascades is British Columbia. That's because the North Cascades are *in* British Columbia. They extend across the imaginary line dividing the U.S. from Canada.

That doesn't mean the four Canadian trips in this book are mere geopolitical tokens. They're in the book because they're stellar. Only when you've hiked them have you sampled the best the range has to offer.

And the best hiking the North Cascades offers is, in our opinion, the equal of any on earth.

TRIPS AT A GLANCE *Trips in each category are listed according to geographic location: starting in the north and moving roughly from west to east, then south. After the trip name, the round-trip distance is listed, followed by the elevation gain.*

DAYHIKES AT A GLANCE

1	First Brother Mountain	13.6 mi (22 km)	2680 ft (817 m)
2	Red Mountain	8.1 mi (13 km)	1640 ft (500 m)
3	Stone City	8.2 mi (13.2 km)	2730 ft (832 m)
4	Lakeview Mountain	10 mi (16.1 km)	3228 ft (984 m)
5	Heliotrope Ridge	6.5 mi (10.5 km)	1900 ft (580 m)
6	Skyline Divide	10 mi (16.1 km)	2163 ft (659 m)
7	Excelsior Ridge	9 mi (14.5 km)	1780 ft (543 m)
8	Church Mountain	8.4 mi (13.5 km)	3600 ft (1097 m)
9	Yellow Aster Butte	7 mi (11.3 km)	2550 ft (777 m)
10	Mt. Larrabee	10 mi (16.1 km)	2300 ft (701 m)
11	Goat Mountain	8.4 mi (13.5 km)	2950 ft (899 m)
12	Hannegan Peak	10 mi (16.1 km)	3086 ft (941 m)
13	Table Mountain	3 mi (5 km)	600 ft (183 m)
14	Ptarmigan Ridge	9.4 mi (15.1 km)	1000 ft (305 m)
15	Lake Ann	8.2 mi (13.2 km)	1700 ft (518 m)
16	Rainbow Ridge	4.4 mi (7.1 km)	1200 ft (366 m)
17	Railroad Grade	8 mi (12.9 km)	2900 ft (884 m)
18	Scott Paul	7.9 mi (12.7 km)	1800 ft (550 m)
19	Trappers Peak	10.6 mi (17.1 km)	3364 ft (1025 m)
20	Sourdough Mountain	11 mi (17.7 km)	5085 ft (1550 m)
21	Fourth of July Pass	11.4 mi (18.3 km)	2880 ft (878 m)
22	Easy Pass	7.2 mi (11.6 km)	2800 ft (853 m)
23	Heather & Maple passes	7.2 mi (11.6 km)	1995 ft (608 m)
24	Cutthroat Pass	10 mi (16.1 km)	2000 ft (610 m)
25	Blue Lake	4.4 mi (7.1 km)	1100 ft (335 m)
26	Windy Pass	7.4 mi (11.9 km)	1000 ft (305 m)
27	Grasshopper Pass	11 mi (17.7 km)	2000 ft (610 m)
28	Silver Lake	9.2 mi (14.8 km)	1800 ft (549 m)
29	Hidden Lake Peaks Lookout	9 mi (14.5 km)	3200 ft (975 m)
30	Boston Basin	8 mi (12.9 km)	3000 ft (914 m)
31	Cascade Pass	7.4 mi (11.9 km)	1800 ft (549 m)
32	Tiffany Mountain	6 mi (9.7 km)	1742 ft (531 m)
33	Stilleto Lake	10.4 mi (16.7 km)	3100 ft (945 m)
34	Green Mountain	8 mi (12.9 km)	3000 ft (914 m)
35	Lake Twentytwo	5.4 mi (8.7 km)	1313 ft (400 m)
36	Mt. Dickerman	8.6 mi (13.8 km)	3923 ft (1196 m)

37	Goat Lake	10.4 mi (16.7 km)	1261 ft (384 m)
38	Gothic Basin	9.4 mi (15.1 km)	2639 ft (804 m)
39	Blanca Lake	8 mi (12.9 km)	3328 ft (1015 m)
40	Spider Gap	16.4 mi (26.4 km)	3600 ft (1097 m)

BACKPACK TRIPS AT A GLANCE

41	Horseshoe Basin	13 mi (21 km)	1200 ft (366 m)
42	Whatcom Pass	45 mi (72.4 km)	10,000 ft (3048 m)
43	Park Creek Pass	40.1 mi (64.5 km)	8840 ft (2694 m)
44	Image Lake	33.6 mi (54.1 km)	4300 ft (1311 m)
45	Lake Byrne	21.4 mi (34.4 km)	5060 ft (1542 m)
46	Pilot Ridge / White Pass	29.1 mi (46.8 km)	6000 ft (1830 m)
47	Buck Creek Pass	19.2 mi (31 km)	3100 ft (945 m)
48	Pyramid Mountain	18.4 mi (29.6 km)	3900 ft (1189 m)
49	Lyman Lake	18.6 mi (30 km)	2398 ft (731 m)
50	Lake Chelan	17 mi (27.4 km)	2200 ft (671 m)

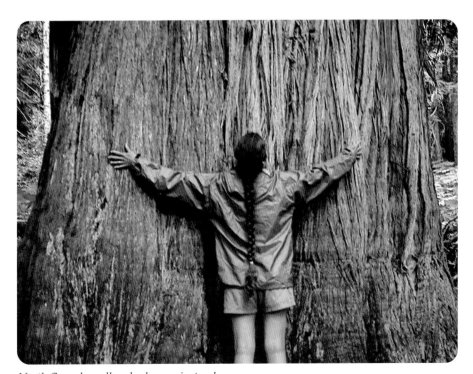

North Cascades valleys harbor ancient cedars.

SHOULDER-SEASON TRIPS

Shoulder-season is a travel-industry term referring to the months before and after the popular, main season. We use it to describe early-summer and late-fall trips that allow you to start hiking by mid-May, and continue hiking perhaps into November. Low elevation or sun exposure ensures these trails are snow-free sooner and longer than others. You'll generally be hiking through forest, but hey, you'll be hiking.

These five trips are designated *Shoulder Season* in the text:

Goat Mountain (11), **Fourth of July Pass (21)**, **Lake Twentytwo (35)**, **Goat Lake (37)**, and **Lake Chelan (50)**.

All are dayhikes except Lake Chelan, which is primarily a backpack trip, though dayhiking a section of it is certainly possible.

The other shoulder-season backpacking options are not labeled as such in the text, because only in summer is it possible to hike them completely. But in spring or fall you can backpack their lower reaches through glorious, ancient forest:

43 Park Creek Pass Initial section: upstream along Thunder Creek, as far as Tricouni camp.

44 Image Lake Initial section: upstream along the Suiattle River, past Canyon Creek to the 10.8-mi (17.4-km) fork.

46 Pilot Ridge / White Pass Final section, in reverse: upstream along the North Fork Sauk River, as far as McKinaw shelter.

MAPS

Since the early 1990s, we've hiked nearly 2,000 mi (3,220 km) in the North Cascades. Green Trails maps have been with us every step of the way, and they've been our primary reference while writing this book.

They're the best topographic maps available for the range. They're easy to read. They clearly mark all the trails in green ink. They state the significant elevations. They even indicate the distances between major junctions. We highly recommend Green Trails maps (www.greentrailsmaps.com).

The maps we created and that accompany each trip in this book are for general orientation only. Our *On Foot* directions are extremely detailed, so refering to a topo map shouldn't be necessary. But if you want to take one with you, buy the Green Trails map/s listed in the stats box for the trail you'll be hiking.

Carrying a topo map is a safety measure, of course, but you're sure to appreciate it for other reasons: (1) If the terrain through which you're hiking intrigues you, a topo map will enrich your experience. (2) After reaching a summit, a topo map will enable you to interpret the surrounding geography. (3) On a long, rough hike, a topo map will make it even easier to follow our directions.

Should you want a single, large map showing most of the area covered in this book, we recommend the Trails Illustrated North Cascades National Park Trail Map published by National Geographic (www.ngmapstore.com). It's printed on waterproof, tear-resistant material with a durable plastic coating.

Green Trails does not offer maps for the four Canadian trips covered in this book. You can, however, download maps for these trips free-of-charge by visiting www.bcparks.ca, then clicking on (1) "find a park," (2) "m" for Manning Provincial Park, or "c" for Cathedral Provincial Park, (3) "map / brochure," and (4) "park map."

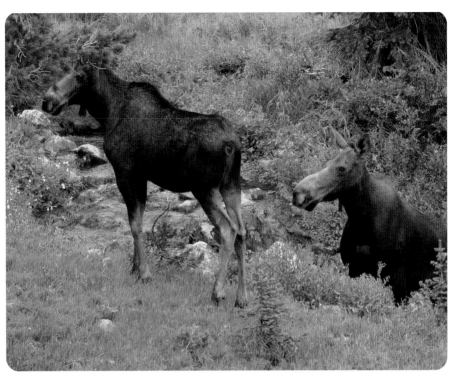

Watch for moose in wet areas.

CARRY A COMPASS

Left and *right* are relative. Any hiking guidebook relying solely on these inadequate and potentially misleading terms should be shredded and dropped into a recycling bin.

You'll find all the *On Foot* descriptions in this book include frequent compass directions. That's the only way to accurately, reliably guide a hiker.

What about GPS? Compared to a compass, GPS units are heavier, bulkier, more fragile, more complex, more time consuming, occasionally foiled by vegetation or topography, dependent on batteries, and way more expensive.

Keep in mind that the compass directions provided in this book are of use only if you're carrying a compass. Granted, our route descriptions are so detailed, you'll rarely have to check your compass. But bring one anyway, just in case. A compass is required hiking equipment—anytime, anywhere, regardless of your level of experience, or your familiarity with the terrain.

Clip your compass to the shoulder strap of your pack, so you can glance at it quickly and easily. Even if you never have to rely on your compass, occasionally checking it will strengthen your sense of direction—an enjoyable, helpful, and conceivably lifesaving asset.

Keep in mind that our stated compass directions are always in reference to true north. In the North Cascades, that's approximately 18.5° left of (counterclockwise from) magnetic north. If that puzzles, you, read your compass owner's manual.

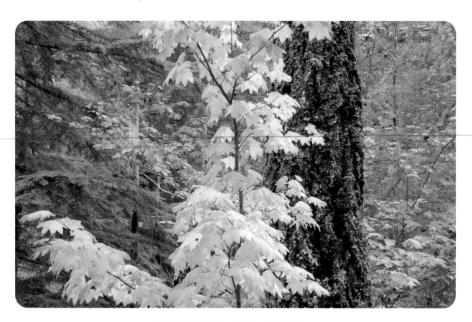

PHYSICAL CAPABILITY

Until you gain experience judging your physical capability and that of your companions, these guidelines might be helpful. Anything longer than a 7-mi (11-km) round-trip day hike can be very taxing for someone who doesn't hike regularly. A 1400-ft (425-m) elevation gain in that distance is challenging but possible for anyone in average physical condition. Very fit hikers are comfortable hiking 11 mi (18 km) and ascending 3100 ft (950 ft)—or more—in a single day.

Backpacking 11 mi (18 km) in two days is a reasonable goal for most beginners. Hikers who backpack a couple times a season can enjoyably manage 17 mi (27 km) in two days. Avid backpackers should find 24 mi (34 km) in two days no problem. On three- to five-day trips, a typical backpacker prefers not to push beyond 10 mi (16 km) a day. Remember: it's always safer to underestimate your limits.

LEAVE YOUR ITINERARY

Even if you're hiking in a group, and especially if you're going solo, it's prudent to leave your itinerary in writing with a reliable family member or friend. Agree on precisely when they should alert the authorities if you have not returned or called. Be sure to follow through. Forgetting to tell your contact person you've safely completed your trip could result in an unnecessary, expensive search. You wouldn't want to be billed for that. Nor would you want a rescue team risking their lives, combing the wilds trying to find you, while you're actually safe, in the bosom of civilization.

WILDERNESS ETHICS

We hope you're already conscientious about respecting nature and other people. If not, here's how to pay off some of your karmic debt load.

Let wildflowers live. They blossom for only a few fleeting weeks.

Uprooting them doesn't enhance your enjoyment, and it prevents others from seeing them at all. We once heard parents urge a string of children to pick as many different-colored flowers as they could find. Great. Teach kids to entertain themselves by destroying nature, so the world continues marching toward environmental collapse.

Stay on the trail. Shortcutting causes erosion. It doesn't save time on steep ascents, because you'll soon be slowing to catch your breath. On a steep descent, it increases the likelihood of injury. When hiking cross-country in a group, soften your impact by spreading out.

Roam meadows with your eyes, not your boots. Again, stay on the trail. If it's braided, follow the main path. When you're compelled to take a photo among wildflowers, try to walk on rocks.

Leave no trace. Be aware of your impact. Travel lightly on the land. At campgrounds, limit your activity to areas already denuded. After a rest stop, and especially after camping, take a few minutes to look for and obscure any evidence of your stay. Restore the area to its natural state. Remember: tents can leave scars. Pitch yours on an existing tentsite whenever possible. If none is available, choose a patch of dirt, gravel, pine needles, or maybe a dried-up tarn. Never pitch your tent on grass, no matter how appealing it looks. If you do, and others follow, the grass will soon be gone.

Avoid building fires. Prohibited in many backcountry areas, they're a luxury not a necessity. Don't plan to cook over a fire; it's inefficient and wasteful. If you pack food that requires cooking, bring a stove. If you must indulge in a campfire, keep it small. Use the metal firebox if one is provided, or an existing fire ring made of rocks. If there are no boxes or rings, build your fire on mineral soil or gravel, not in the organic layer. Never scorch meadows. Below a stream's high-water line is best. Garbage with metal or plastic content will not burn; pack it all out. Limit your wood gathering to deadfall about the size of your forearm. Wood that requires effort (breaking, chopping, dragging) is part of the scenery; let it be. After thoroughly dousing your fire, dismantle the fire ring and scatter the ashes. Keep in mind that untended and unextinguished campfires are the prime causes of forest fires.

Be quiet at backcountry campsites. Most of us are out there to enjoy tranquility. If you want to party, go to a bar.

Pack out everything you bring. Never leave a scrap of trash anywhere. This includes toilet paper, nut shells, even cigarette butts. People who drop butts in the wilderness are buttheads. They're buttheads in the city too, but it's worse in the wilds. Fruit peels are also trash. They take years to decompose, and wild animals won't eat them. If you bring fruit on your hike, you're responsible for the peels. And don't just pack out *your* trash. Leave nothing behind, whether you brought it or not. Clean up behind others. Don't be hesitant or oblivious. Be proud. Keep a small plastic bag handy, so picking up trash will be a habit instead of a pain. It's infuriating and disgusting to see what people toss on the trail. Often the tossing is mindless, but sometimes it's intentional. Anyone who leaves a pile of toilet paper and unburied feces deserves to have their nose rubbed in it.

Poop without impact. Use the outhouses at trailheads and campgrounds whenever possible. Don't count on them being stocked with toilet paper; always pack your own in a plastic bag. If you know there's a campground ahead, try to wait until you get there.

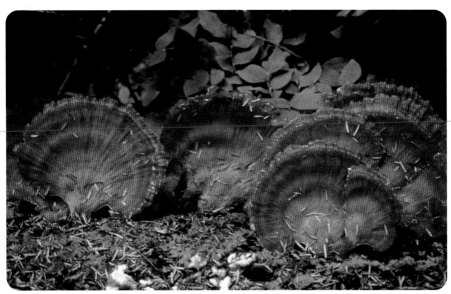

Chicken of the Forest

In the wilds, choose a site at least 66 yd (60 m) from trails and water sources. Ground that receives sunlight part of the day is best. Use a trowel to dig a small cat hole—4 to 8 inches (10 to 20 cm) deep, 4 to 6 inches (10 to 15 cm) wide—in soft, dark, biologically active soil. Afterward, throw a handful of dirt into the hole, stir with a stick to speed decomposition, replace your diggings, then camouflage the site. Pack out used toilet paper in a plastic bag. You can drop the paper (not the plastic) in the next outhouse you pass. Always clean your hands with a moisturizing hand sanitizer, like Purell. Carry enough for the entire trip. Sold in drugstores, it comes in conveniently small, lightweight, plastic bottles.

Urinate off trail, well away from water sources and tentsites. The salt in urine attracts animals. They'll defoliate urine-soaked vegetation, so aim for dirt or pine needles.

Keep streams and lakes pristine. When brushing your teeth or washing dishes, do it well away from water sources and tentsites. Use only biodegradable soap. Carry water far enough so the waste water will percolate through soil and break down without directly polluting the wilderness water. Scatter waste water widely. Even biodegradable soap is a pollutant; keep it out of streams and lakes. On short backpack trips, you shouldn't need to wash clothes or yourself. If necessary, rinse your clothes or splash yourself off—without soap.

Respect the reverie of other hikers. On busy trails, don't feel it's necessary to communicate with everyone you pass. Most of us are seeking solitude, not a soiree. A simple greeting is sufficient to convey good will. Obviously, only you can judge what's appropriate at the time. But it's usually presumptuous and annoying to blurt out advice without being asked. "Boy, have you got a long way to go." "The views are much better up there." "Be careful, it gets rougher." If anyone wants to know, they'll ask. Some people are sly. They start by asking where you're going, so they can tell you all about it. Offer

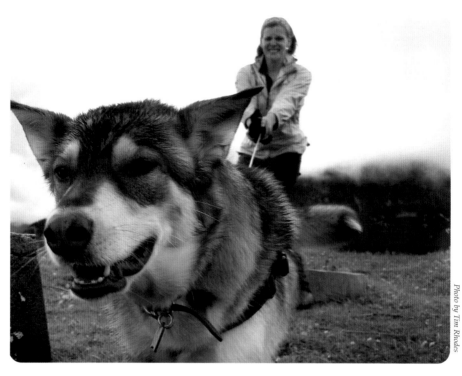

Photo by Tim Rhodes

unsolicited information only to warn other hikers about conditions ahead that could seriously affect their trip.

HIKING WITH YOUR DOG

Dogs are prohibited within North Cascades National Park. As for the other jurisdictions within the area covered by this book, national recreation areas allow leashed dogs on most trails, and wilderness areas and national forests permit unleashed dogs.

But before you take your dog hiking with you, ask the appropriate authorities about their current, specific policies regarding dogs in the back-country.

Bringing your dog hiking with you, however, isn't simply a matter of "Can I or can't I?" The larger question is "Should I or shouldn't I?"

Consider the social consequences. Most dog owners think their pets are angelic. But other people rarely agree, especially hikers confined overnight in a backcountry campground where someone's brought a dog.

A curious dog, even if friendly, can be a nuisance. A barking dog is annoying. A person continually yelling unheeded commands at a disobedient dog is infuriating, because it amounts to *two* annoying animals, not just one. An untrained dog, despite the owner's hearty reassurance that "he won't hurt you," can be frightening.

Consider your environmental responsibilities. Many dog owners blithely allow their pets to pollute streams and lakes, or foul campgrounds. The fact that their dog is crapping in the trail doesn't occur to them, but it certainly does to the next hiker who comes along and steps in it.

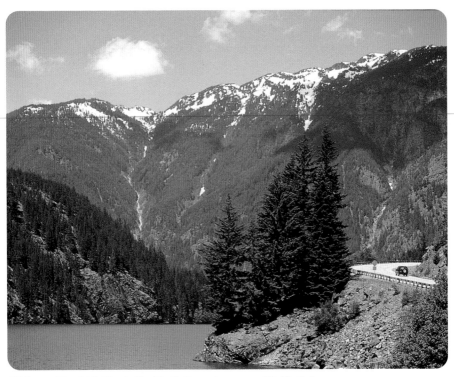

Highway 20, which bisects the North Cascades, passes Diablo Lake.

Consider the safety issues. Dogs in the backcountry are a danger to themselves. For example, porcupines prowling campgrounds at night are likely to spike them. Even worse, they can endanger their owners and other hikers, because dogs infuriate bears. If a dog runs off, it might reel a bear back with it.

This isn't a warning not to bring your dog. We've completed lengthy backpack trips with friends whose dogs we enjoyed immensely. This is a plea to see your dog objectively, from the perspective of your fellow hikers.

WHO'S IN CHARGE AROUND HERE?

The North Cascades comprise four distinct land jurisdictions: national park, national recreation areas, wilderness areas, and unprotected areas in national forest.

The mandate of **North Cascades National Park** is to protect the wilderness quality. Removing rocks and picking wildflowers are prohibited. Dogs and other pets are not allowed on trails—only on roads, and then only on a leash. Fishing is allowed, but you must have a license. Hunting is illegal.

National Recreation Areas allow more tourist development and permit leashed dogs on most trails and horses on some. Hunting and mining are prohibited.

Wilderness Areas are supposed to be preserved in their wild state. Dogs, horseback riding, hunting, and fishing are allowed. New roads, mechanized equipment, commercial development, even mountain bikes are prohibited. Mining is permitted on some patented claims, but only after the Forest Service has conducted an impact study and elicited public response.

Multiple-use is the key principle governing **National Forests**. Along with mining, logging, and commercial development, many forms of recreation are allowed, including mountain biking and motorcycle riding on some trails. Dogs are also permitted. But wilderness areas within national forests have the same limitations outlined above.

Read the *Backcountry Permits* section for details about camping in the national park and national recreation areas. Permits are not necessary elsewhere. In wilderness areas, rangers strongly urge you to camp only in designated campsites, although it's not a legal requirement. You can camp anywhere you want in national forests, but a lack of restrictions doesn't relieve you of responsibility. Always follow leave-no-trace camping practices.

BACKCOUNTRY PERMITS

Backpackers entering North Cascades National Park, Ross Lake National Recreation Area, or Lake Chelan National Recreation Area, must have a backcountry camping permit. Permits are free of charge. But you can obtain them only in person, either the day you intend to start your trip or the day before, no earlier. First come, first served. You cannot make reservations.

The North Cascades National Park Wilderness Information Center in Marblemount is the best place to get a permit. It offers the most current and comprehensive information on backcountry conditions. Other offices that issue permits are the North Cascades National Park Headquarters in Sedro-Woolley, the Glacier Public Service Center, the North Cascades Visitor Center in Newhalem, the Methow Valley Visitor Center in Winthrop, the Chelan Ranger Station, and the Golden West Visitor Center in Stehekin.

At some of the above locations, after-hours self-registration is allowed. For these and other details, visit www.nps.gov/noca (click on "plan your visit," then "wilderness trip planner," then "backcountry permits"), or phone the National Park Headquarters in Sedro-Woolley: (360) 856-5700 ext. 515.

Only with a permit in hand is your site at an official backcountry campground reserved. Camping elsewhere is prohibited, unless you get a permit for cross-country camping (1 mi / 1.6 km outside an official campground, 0.5 mi / 0.8 km off trail, and 200 ft / 60 m from water). Even cross-country camping is restricted to certain areas—usually brush-choked drainages—so doing it properly can be a challenge. If you try it, allow an extra couple hours of daylight to establish camp.

Permits are a pain. Request one in midseason for a popular area—Copper Ridge, for example—and you might find the campgrounds you want to stay at are full. This means adjusting your itinerary—hiking shorter or longer days than you'd prefer—to ensure you end up at a campground with an available site. Sticking to an itinerary, even a reasonable one, can be difficult in the backcountry. After all, once you leave the trailhead, you're on an adventure. Adventures, by definition, never fit neatly into rigid schedules. Besides, one of the joys of wilderness travel should be walking away from the constraints of modern civilization.

For the permit system to work, every hiker must adhere to it, and they don't. Many simply fall off schedule. Some change plans en route. Others just ignore the permit requirement from the outset. We've pitched our tent at backcountry campgrounds where none of the campers, us included, was sleeping where our permits said we should be.

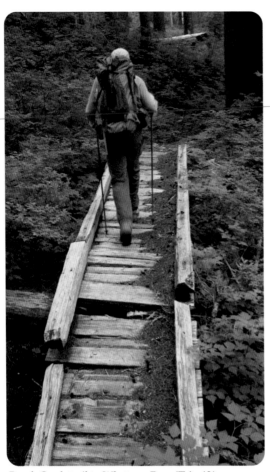

Brush Creek trail to Whatcom Pass (Trip 42)

So, just because you have a permit, don't assume an empty campsite is awaiting your arrival. You might have to make friends with other backpackers and share a site. Be reasonable and flexible. If at all possible, camp only according to your permit. Keep in mind, if a ranger catches you camping illegally you'll be severely lectured and possibly fined. And never let your frustration with the permit system be an excuse for damaging the fragile mountain environment. Always follow leave-no-trace practices.

The permit system is intended to ensure you enjoy a tranquil camping experience, and to protect the wilderness from the effects of an ever-increasing number of visitors. It's hypocritical to be part of the problem, yet not participate in the solution. For that reason alone, the system deserves our respect and cooperation.

NORTHWEST FOREST PASS

To park your vehicle at National Forest trailheads in Washington and Oregon, you must have a Northwest Forest Pass. Pass sales generate millions of dollars each year. At least 80% of the total (up to a maximum of 95%) comes back to you in the form of maintenance and improvement of trailheads, trails and campgrounds. As a result, the Forest Service now serves hikers in myriad ways that its shrinking budget previously did not allow. You can purchase a day pass or an annual pass. They're sold at Forest Service offices (see page 253).

You can buy your pass online from the Washington Trails Association (www.wta.org). You'll find "forest passes" under "store" on their home-page menu. All WTA membership packages (also under "store" on their home-page menu) include annual passes. In return for two days' volunteer trail-work with WTA, they'll give you an annual pass at no charge. See "trail work" on their home-page menu.

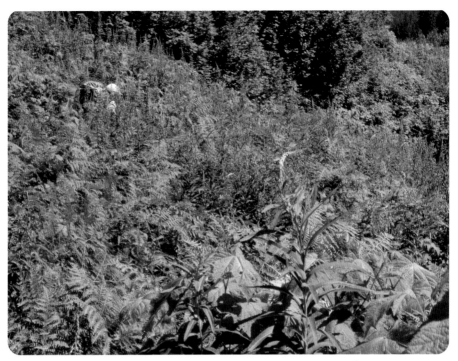

Tall, thick brush en route to Whatcom Pass (Trip 42). Note hiker, upper left.

VOLUNTEER TRAIL MAINTENANCE

It's the brush and deadfall that need cutting, not the Forest Service trail-work budget. But it always seems to be the other way around.

North Cascades trails need constant maintenance. The moist, temperate climate spawns brush so luxuriant it can obscure a path in a single summer. Steep slopes and heavy rainfall result in frequent, sometimes massive erosion. Dense forests = lots of deadfall.

Plus, many trails weren't constructed. They were boot-built by miners and climbers. Miners were obsessed with getting rich, not with providing recreation opportunities. Climbers likewise had no regard for who followed them. Their hurry-scurry routes deteriorate rapidly.

Legislators think cutbacks merely prevent construction of new trails, which they consider unnecessary. They don't realize funds are required just to keep existing trails walkable.

Forget about new trails. In the North Cascades, we're losing the ones we have. Which is why hikers need to give—a little time, a little money, maybe a little of both.

The Washington Trails Association schedules frequent work parties, and you're invited. It's hard labor, but all they ask is a single day.

Take one of your summer Saturdays, and instead of bashing through the obstacles, devote it to clearing them, so hiking becomes more enjoyable for everyone.

Volunteer trail maintenance is also a great way to meet spirited people who share your interests. Visit www.wta.org to learn more.

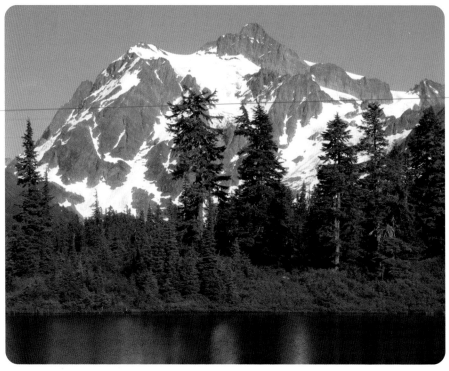

Mt. Shuksan, from Picture Lake, Highway 542

CASCADIAN CLIMATE

The volatile North Cascades climate will have you building shrines to placate the weather gods. Conditions change quickly and dramatically.

Storms roll in off the Pacific Ocean, unleashing heavy precipitation on the west side of the range but leaving the drier east side thirsty. On the west, it seems to rain half the time during summer. Even many rain-free days are cloudy. So don't squander a blue sky. Celebrate it, by hiking fast and far. When it's socked-in and pouring on the west, however, there's a chance it's merely overcast and pleasantly cool farther east. So don't surrender to the weather. Change it, by driving over the crest.

Summers are hot throughout the range. Daytime temperatures average 75° F (24° C) on the west, 85° F (29.5° C) on the east. The mercury can soar as high 90° F (32° C) on the west, higher on the east. Avoid the worst heat by hiking early or late in the day. You'll find only slight relief at higher elevations or in deep forest.

Though the sun is often tempered somewhat on the west side by abundant clouds and shade, consistently high humidity makes the heat oppressive nonetheless. But the east side, despite low humidity, is even worse in summer and best avoided. It's a furnace. Clear skies and sparser forests make it difficult to find relief from the sun. Those same qualities, however, make the east side attractive for spring and fall hiking.

By late June, there's usually been enough warm weather and subsequent snowmelt that your dayhiking options are numerous. The snowline should be near 6500 ft (1980 m) on north slopes then, and near 5500 ft (1676 m) on south slopes. Just one week of clear, sunny weather greatly increases trail accessibility.

The crux of most long backpack trips probably won't be safely passable until mid July, unless you're competent with an ice axe.

Snowstorms can hit the first week of September. An early wave of cold and snow, however, is often followed by warm days into mid-October. But the days are shorter then and the nights colder, so backpacking isn't as pleasant. Fall colors usually reach full intensity by late September.

Typically, the Cascadian climate will grant you about three months of high-country hiking. That's just 25% of the year. Carpe diem.

SCOURGE OF THE CASCADES

You'll be tired, sweaty, thirsty. You'll stop for a rest. Within seconds, they'll be all over you: fingernail sized, crunchy-to-the-touch, black flies.

Dozens will assault your legs, attack your arms, land on your neck, strafe your ears, crawl up your nose. And if you don't swat them, you'll feel the sudden, sharp prick of their vicious bite.

Because they're sluggish, you'll easily kill many. Whap. Whap. Whap. But they're impossible to vanquish. They just keep coming. For every one you swat, three more appear. So you gulp a few sips of water and move on. Perpetual motion is your best defense. But there are other tactics you'll find helpful.

Black flies, as well as the larger deerflies and horseflies, become a nuisance in the North Cascades every year around late July. If the weather's been hot, they'll harass you by mid-July. The blitz will continue until the weather cools, probably in September.

Mosquitoes are bothersome here too, of course, but no more so than in most mountain ranges. Except in the North Cascades' most notoriously mosquito-infested areas, like the Lyman Lakes basin, it's the flies that will torment you.

Mid-summer, when the flies are worst, begin long hikes very early. Rising temperature rouses flies. When the sun's heat penetrates the forest—about 9 a.m.—it's as if the flies hear their starting gun. Cooler temperatures subdue them, so consider starting backpack trips or very short day-hikes after 4 p.m.

Citronella bug repellent or eucalyptus oil deters flies from biting but doesn't actually disperse them. They'll still swarm. Repellents containing DEET repel them, but it's poisonous. We prefer body armor: long pants, and a loose, lightweight, longsleeve shirt. We make rest stops and mealtime more tolerable by donning head nets made of fine, nylon mesh.

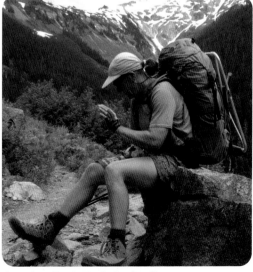

Swatting flies in Ruth Creek valley

Wearing a head net while hiking, however, obscures your vision and can be uncomfortably hot. For a superior anti-fly shield while in motion, tuck a bandana under your hat. Let it drape, Lawrence-of-Arabia style, over your ears, temples, cheeks and neck. If you don't carry trekking poles, it's less tiring to wave a bandana around your head and legs than it is to flap your arms.

The fly population is thinner at higher elevations. A stiff breeze keeps them grounded, same as mosquitoes. So you can look forward to relief at most passes. But it's easy to go berserk before you get there, if the flies are bad below.

Adopt the temperament of a Zen Buddhist monk. Refuse to be enraged by the pests. Observe them. Appreciate how slow and unintelligent they are. Imagine speedy, clever flies. Now *that* would be a truly diabolical torture.

BATTLING BRUSH

Brush is a defining characteristic of North Cascades valleys and alpine slopes. The term *brush* refers to all the shrubs, bushes, sedges, and grasses that grow rapidly and profusely in this temperate range.

Hiking a brushy trail is discouraging for all but machete-minded commandos. It obscures the tread, impeding your balance and speed. It scratches your arms and claws at your legs. If the brush is wet, whatever you're wearing will soon be sodden. Stinging nettles make your skin itch. Devil's Club has fangs so savagely sharp they seem almost carnivorous.

Brush is also a verb meaning *to cut and clear*. Some trails become choked with vegetation unless they're brushed annually by a work crew. Volunteers are critically needed in this effort. See the *Volunteer Trail Maintenance* section.

If someone wielding hedge clippers—paid or volunteer—hasn't brushed the trail you're hiking before your arrival, be prepared to gird your loins. Tall gaiters are helpful, and they repel water, but they leave your knees and thighs exposed. Your best defense is to wear a pair of long pants. If the brush is really high, break out the heavy artillery: your longsleeve shirt.

COUGARS

You'll probably never see a cougar. But they live in the North Cascades, and they can be dangerous, so you should know a bit about them.

Elsewhere referred to as a puma, mountain lion, or panther, the cougar is an enormous, graceful cat. An adult male can reach the size of a big human: 175 lb (80 kg), and 8 ft (2.4 m) long including a 3-ft (1-m) tail. In the North Cascades, they tend to be a tawny grey.

Nocturnal, secretive, solitary creatures, cougars come together only to mate. Each cat establishes a territory of 125 to 175 sq mi (200 to 280 sq km). They favor dense forest that provides cover while hunting. They also hide among rock outcroppings and in steep canyons.

Habitat loss and aggressive predator-control programs have severely limited the range of this mysterious animal that once lived throughout North America. Still, cougars are not considered endangered or threatened. In Washington they're listed as a game animal and are hunted. Two other, smaller cats roam the North Cascades: lynx and bobcat.

Cougars are carnivores. They eat everything from mice to elk but prefer deer. They occasionally stalk people but rarely attack them. In folklore, cougars are called *ghost cats* or *ghost walkers*, for good reason. They're very shy and typically avoid human contact. Nevertheless, cougars have attacked solo hikers and lone cross-country skiers.

Cougar sightings and encounters are increasing due to a thriving cougar population, humanity's ever-expanding footprint, and the growing number of people visiting the wilderness.

If you're lucky enough to see a cougar, treasure the experience. Just remember they're unpredictable. Follow these suggestions:

• Never hike alone in areas of known cougar sightings. Keep children close to you; pick them up if you see fresh cougar scat or tracks.

• Never approach a cougar, especially a feeding one. Never flee from a cougar, or even turn your back on it. Sudden movement might trigger an instinctive attack. Avert your gaze and speak to it in a calm, soothing voice. Hold your ground or back away slowly. Always give the animal a way out.

• If a cougar approaches, spread your arms, open your jacket, do anything you can to enlarge your image. If it acts aggressively, wave your arms, shout, throw rocks or sticks. If attacked, fight back. Don't play dead.

BEARS

Bears are not a problem in the North Cascades, but oblivious hikers are. Too many people are unaware that these mountains support a healthy population of bears. Unprepared for a bear encounter, and ignorant of how to prevent one, they make bears a more serious threat—to themselves and everyone else.

If you're ready for a bear encounter and know how to prevent one, you can hike confidently, secure in the understanding that bears pose little threat.

Black bears are by far the most common species in the North Cascades. There are grizzly bears here as well, but not many. Grizzlies are the slowest reproducing land animals in North America. Only the musk ox is slower. So the North Cascades' grizzly population will remain small. You're unlikely to see a grizzly here. There's a reasonable chance you'll see a black bear.

Grizzlies and blacks can be difficult for an inexperienced observer to tell apart. Both species range in colour from nearly white to cinnamon to black. Full-grown grizzlies are much bigger, but a young grizzly can resemble an adult black bear, so size is not a good indicator. The most obvious differences are that grizzlies have a dished face; a big, muscular shoulder hump; and long, curved front claws. Blacks have a straight face; no hump; and shorter, less visible front claws. Grizzlies are potentially more dangerous than black bears, although a black bear sow with cubs can be just as aggressive. Be wary of all bears.

Any bear might attack when surprised. If you're hiking, and forest or brush limits your visibility, you can prevent surprising a bear by making noise. Bears hear about as well as humans. Most are as anxious to avoid an encounter as you are. If you warn them of your presence before they see you, they'll usually clear out. So use the most effective noisemaker: your voice. Shout loudly. Keep it up. Don't be embarrassed. Be safe. Yell louder near streams, so your voice carries over the competing noise. Sound off more frequently when hiking into the wind. That's when bears are least able to hear or smell you coming. To learn more, download the *Bears Beware!* MP3 at hikingcamping.com.

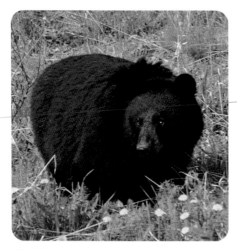

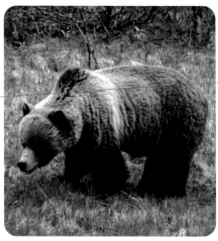

Black bear   *Grizzly bear*

Bears' strongest sense is smell. They can detect an animal carcass several miles away. So keep your pack, tent and campsite odor-free. Double- or triple-wrap all your food in plastic bags. Avoid smelly foods, especially meat and fish. On short backpack trips, consider eating only fresh foods that require no cooking or cleanup. If you cook, do it as far as possible from where you'll be sleeping. Never cook in or near your tent; the fabric might retain odor. Use as few pots and dishes as you can get by with. Be fastidious when you wash them. At night, hang all your food, trash, and anything else that smells (cooking gear, sunscreen, bug repellent, toothpaste, lip balm) in a tree, out of bears' reach. Bring a sturdy stuffsack to serve as your bear bag. Hoist it at least 5 yd/m off the ground and 1.5 yd/m from the tree trunk or other branches. You'll need about 12 yd/m of light nylon cord. Clip the sack to the cord with an ultralight carabiner.

Backpackers who don't properly hang their food at night are inviting bears into their campsite, greatly increasing the chance of a dangerous encounter. And bears are smart. They quickly learn to associate a particular place, or people in general, with an easy meal. They become habituated and lose their fear of man. A habituated bear is a menace to any hiker within its range.

If you see a bear, don't look it in the eyes; it might think you're challenging it. Never run. Initially be still. If you must move, do it in slow motion. Bears are more likely to attack if you flee, and they're fast, much faster than humans. A grizzly can outsprint a racehorse. And it's a myth that bears can't run downhill. They're also strong swimmers. Despite their ungainly appearance, they're excellent climbers too. Still, climbing a tree can be an option for escaping an aggressive bear. Some people have saved their lives this way. Others have been caught in the process. To be out of reach of an adult bear, you must climb at least 10 yd/m very quickly, something few people are capable of. It's generally best to avoid provoking an attack by staying calm, initially standing your ground, making soothing sounds to convey a nonthreatening presence, then retreating slowly.

What should you do when a bear charges? If you're certain it's a lone black bear—not a sow with cubs, not a grizzly—fighting back might be effective. If it's a grizzly, and contact seems imminent, lie face down, with your legs apart and your hands clasped behind your neck. This is safer than the fetal position, which used to be recommended, because it makes it harder for the bear to flip you over. If you play dead, a grizzly is likely to break off the attack once it feels you're no longer a threat. Don't move until you're sure the bear has left the area, then slowly, quietly, get up and walk away. Keep moving, but don't run.

Arm yourself with pepper spray as a last defense. Keep it in a holster, on your hip belt or shoulder strap, where you can grab it fast. Many people have successfully used it to turn back charging bears. Cayenne pepper, highly irritating to a bear's sensitive nose, is the active ingredient. Without causing permanent injury, it disables the bear long enough to let you escape. But vigilance and noise making should prevent you from ever having to spray. Do so only if you really think your life is at risk. You can buy pepper spray at outdoor stores. Counter Assault is a reputable brand.

Remember that your safety is not the only important consideration. Bears themselves are at risk when confronted by people. Whenever bears act aggressively, they're following their natural instinct for self preservation. Often they're protecting their cubs or a food source. Yet if they maul a hiker, they're likely to be killed, or captured and moved, by wildlife management officers. Protecting these beautiful, magnificent creatures is a responsibility hikers must accept.

Merrily disregarding bears is foolish and unsafe. Worrying about them is miserable and unnecessary. Everyone occasionally feels afraid when venturing deep into the mountains, but knowledge and awareness can quell fear of bears. Just take the necessary precautions and remain guardedly alert. Experiencing the grandeur of the North Cascades is certainly worth risking the remote possibility of a bear encounter.

LIGHTNING

Many of the trails in this book lead to meadows, ridges, and peaks where, during a storm, you could be exposed to lightning.

Storms tend to develop in the afternoon, so you can try to reach alpine destinations early in the day. But it's impossible to always evade violent weather. You hike to commune with nature, the power of which can threaten your safety.

Even if you start under a cloudless, blue sky, you might see ominous, black thunderheads marching toward you a few hours later. Upon reaching a high, airy vantage, you could be forced by an approaching storm to decide if and when you should retreat to safer ground.

The following is a summary of lightning precautions recommended by experts. These are not guaranteed solutions. We offer them merely as suggestions to help you make wise choices and reduce your chance of injury.

If your hair is standing on end, there's electricity in the air around you. A lightning strike could be imminent. Get outa there! That's usually down the mountain, but if there's too much open expanse to traverse, look for closer protection.

A direct lightning strike can kill you. It can cause brain damage, heart failure or third-degree burns. Ground current, from a nearby strike, can severely injure you, causing deep burns and tissue damage. Direct strikes are worse, but ground-current contact is far more common.

Avoid a direct strike by getting off exposed ridges and peaks. Even a few yards (meters) off a ridge is better than on top. Avoid isolated, tall trees. A clump of small trees or an opening in the trees is safer.

Avoid ground current by getting out of stream gullies and away from crevices, lichen patches, or wet, solid-rock surfaces. Loose rock, like talus, is safer.

Look for a low-risk area, near a highpoint at least 10 yd/m higher than you. Crouch near its base, at least 1.5 yd/m from cliffs or walls.

Once you choose a place to wait it out, your goal is to prevent brain or heart damage by stopping an electrical charge from flowing through your whole body. Squat with your boots touching one another. If you have a sleeping pad, put it beneath your boots for insulation. Keep your hands away from rocks. Fold your arms across your chest. Stay at least 10 yd/m from your companions, so if one is hit, another can give cardiopulmonary resuscitation.

Deep caves offer protection. Crouch away from the mouth, at least 1.5 yd/m from the walls. But avoid rock overhangs and shallow depressions, because ground current can jump across them. Lacking a deep cave, you're safer in the low-risk area below a highpoint.

HYPOTHERMIA

Many deaths outdoors involve no obvious injury. "Exposure" is usually cited as the killer, but that's a misleading term. It vaguely refers to conditions that contributed to the death. The actual cause is hypothermia: excessive loss of body heat. It can happen with startling speed, in surprisingly mild weather—often between 30 and 50°F (0 and 10°C). Guard against it vigilantly.

Cool temperatures, wetness (perspiration or rain), wind, or fatigue, usually a combination, sap the body of vital warmth. Hypothermia results when heat loss continues to exceed heat gain. Initial symptoms include chills and shivering. Poor coordination, slurred speech, sluggish thinking, and memory loss are next. Intense shivering then decreases while muscular rigidity increases, accompanied by irrationality, incoherence, even hallucinations. Stupor, blue skin, slowed pulse and respiration, and unconsciousness follow. The heartbeat finally becomes erratic until the victim dies.

Avoid becoming hypothermic by wearing synthetic clothing that wicks moisture away from your skin and insulates when wet. Read *Prepare For Your Hike*, in the back of this book, for a description of clothing and equipment that will help you stay warm and dry. Food fuels your internal fire, so bring more than you think you'll need, including several energy bars for emergencies only.

If you can't stay warm and dry, you must escape the wind and rain. Turn back. Keep moving. Eat snacks. Seek shelter. Do it while you're still mentally and physically capable. Watch others in your party for signs of hypothermia. Victims might resist help at first. Trust the symptoms, not the person. Be insistent. Act immediately.

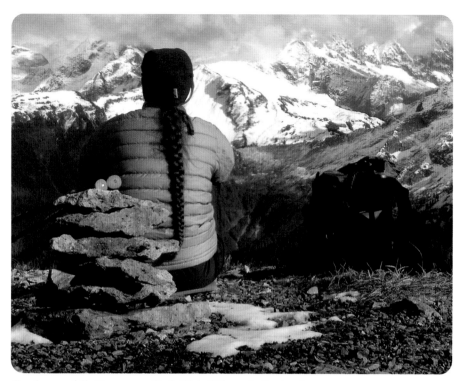

Fresh snowfall, Hannegan Peak (Trip 12), early September

Create the best possible shelter for the victim. Take off his wet clothes and replace them with dry ones. Insulate him from the ground. Provide warmth. A pre-warmed sleeping bag inside a tent is ideal. If necessary, add more warmth by taking off your clothes and getting into the bag with the victim. Build a fire. Keep the victim conscious. Feed him sweets. Carbohydrates quickly convert to heat and energy. In advanced cases, victims should not drink hot liquids.

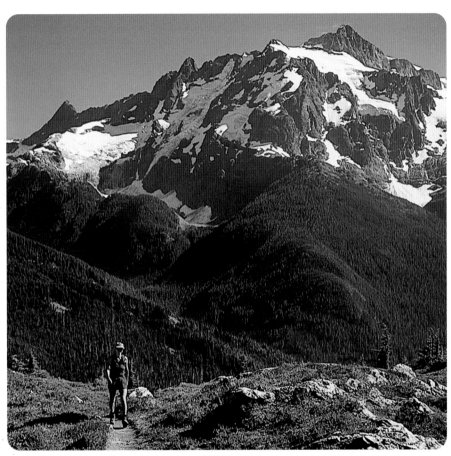

Mt. Shuksan, from Yellow Aster Butte trail (Trip 9)

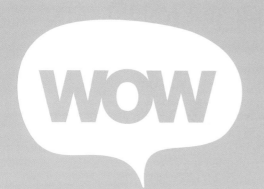

DAYHIKES

TRIP 1
FIRST BROTHER MOUNTAIN

LOCATION	Manning Provincial Park, British Columbia
ROUND TRIP	13.6 mi (22 km) to First Brother Mtn
	26 mi (42 km) to Nicomen Ridge
ELEVATION GAIN	2680 ft (817 m) to First Brother Mtn
	3526 ft (1075 m) to Nicomen Ridge
KEY ELEVATIONS	trailhead 6496 ft (1980 m), Buckhorn camp 5970 ft (1820 m)
	First Brother Mtn 7454 ft (2272 m)
	Nicomen Ridge 6562 ft (2000 m)
HIKING TIME	5½ to 7 hours for First Brother Mtn
	2 days for Nicomen Ridge
DIFFICULTY	easy
MAP	Manning Provincial Park (free download, www.bcparks.ca)

OPINION

Primitive human cultures were sustained by rituals. Today, our rituals are few and shallow. Many of us have none. We think they're unnecessary. But when we go hiking, when we walk the earth and bed down on it, our intention is to live primitively.

So maybe we should begin each hike the way our ancestors began their journeys: with an invocation, a blessing, a ritual that sharpens awareness, heightens appreciation, deepens the experience of whatever lies ahead.

It doesn't have to be lengthy or elaborate. It might be a gesture, or a few whispered words. It can be as simple as ten seconds of silence. Whatever your ritual, an ideal place to inaugurate it would be here, before the langorously long meadow-walk to First Brother Mtn.

The Heather trail, as it's called, traverses a high divide separating rain forest in the west from grassland in the east. It glides through gentle, pastoral meadows where wildflowers grow in painterly profusion.

Hiking here doesn't require the athleticism necessary on many North Cascades trails, so it's more conducive to relaxation, contemplation, meditation—the kind of hiking that allows you to ponder your ritual and its effects.

The challenge you'll face isn't steepness. It's identifying all the blossoms you'll see from mid-July through mid-August. If the previous winter's snowfall was average, and the spring weather has been normal, you can expect a kaleidoscopic floral display, like those that originally inspired the creation of Manning Provincial Park.

In 1931, domestic sheep were overgrazing the area. Citizen protests led to the establishment of Three Brothers Mtn Reserve. In 1941, the meadows plus several thousand hectares of surrounding land were declared a Provincial Park named after E. C. Manning, Chief Forester of British Columbia from 1935 to 1940 and a champion of wilderness preservation.

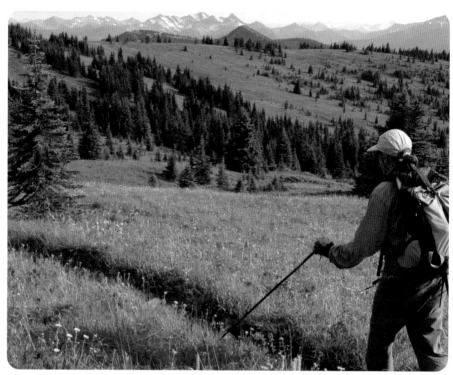

Extensive meadows along the Heather trail

The annual Heather-trail flower show begins in late June. From then until early July, the snowpack rapidly recedes and the groundcover erupts with tiny, white spring-beauties, creamy western anemone, and bright-yellow glacier lilies.

By mid-summer, the variety of form increases, and the array of color explodes. Here are few of the wildflowers you'll likely see:

- orange, crimson, scarlet, or rose Indian paintbrush, as well as the typical vibrant red
- pale cream, pink, or blue lupine, as well as the typical light- to deep-purple
- yellow, subalpine buttercup
- bright-yellow cinquefoil (See photo on page 60.)
- cow parsnip, whose white flowers cluster in a large, flat-topped umbrella at the end of a long stalk
- Indian hellebore, with light-green, accordion-pleated, oblong leaves about 10 inches (22 cm) long. (See photo on page 35.)
- Sitka valerian, whose tiny, white to pale-pink flowers grow atop a high stalk

And there are interesting stories associated with many of these flowers. Sitka valerian, for example, was a popular aphrodisiac among Europeans. According to legend, the Pied Piper attracted followers by stuffing his pockets with it.

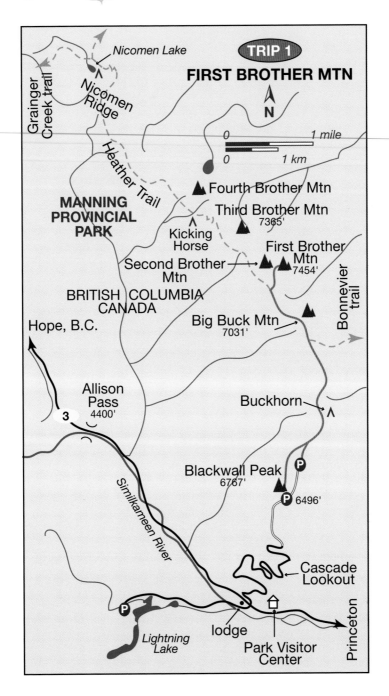

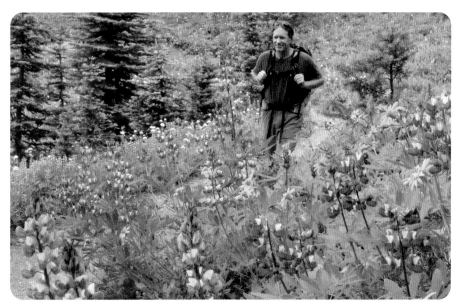

Lupine are profuse along the Heather trail.

As for eyes-up scenery, you'll occasionally gasp at the impressive, white bulk of the North Cascades spanning the southern horizon. But the immediate topography lacks drama. Less than 25,000 years ago, glaciers scoured the tops off the nearby peaks: Big Buck, First, Second, Third, and Fourth Brother mountains. The resulting appearance is more Yellowstone than Pacific Northwest.

The trail's popularity is also Yellowstone-like. Not only are these highland meadows a mere two-and-a-half-hour drive from Vancouver, they're world famous. We've encountered botanical-minded hiking groups here from Great Britain and Germany. The crowd diminishes past Buckhorn camp. Tranquility increases past First Brother Mtn. Solitude is likely five hours from the trailhead, past Kicking Horse camp. Avoid hiking here on weekends.

To mitigate the affects of heavy visitation, B.C. Parks has civilized the Heather trail. Wood chips cover the tread part way. Substantial bridges span even minor streams. Trenches and drainage pipes prevent erosion. Tent platforms protect vegetation. So the enormous *Wilderness Camp* signs are oxymoronic. But this is grizzly-bear country nonetheless, so take all the standard precautions. And bring a stove. Fires are prohibited at Buckhorn and Kicking Horse camps.

The summit of First Brother Mtn is the optimal dayhike destination. Fully savoring the area, however, requires backpacking. One night will suffice. Start early, pitch your tent at Kicking Horse camp, wander out Nicomen Ridge in the afternoon, then exit the next day.

Whatever you do, ignore Buckhorn camp. It's too close to the trailhead to afford peace. And don't be tempted to make this a one-way trip. Turn around at the north end of Nicomen Ridge. If you descend past Nicomen Lake, then follow Grainger Creek and the Skaist River out to Hwy 3, you'll trudge through forest all day and miss repeating one of the greatest meadowland walks in the North Cascades.

FACT

From Hope, British Columbia, drive east on Hwy 5 then Hwy 3 about 42 mi (67 km) to Manning Park Lodge. Turn left (north) onto the road signed for Cascade Lookout. Pavement ends at 3.7 mi (6 km). Reach the trailhead parking lot beneath Blackwall Peak at 9.3 mi (15 km), 6496 ft (1980 m).

The signed Heather trail—initially an old road—leads north. With incidental variation, this will remain your general direction of travel all the way to First Brother Mtn, which is directly north of the trailhead.

Within 15 minutes cross a meadow where paintbrush and lupine are profuse. Big Buck and First Brother mountains are visible north. About 25 minutes from the trailhead, enter a bigger meadow where Indian hellebore dominates.

At 1.2 mi (2 km) reach a junction. Right ascends back to the upper parking lot. Proceed straight, still on a road-width path.

After a 400-ft (125-m) descent through spruce forest, reach **Buckhorn camp** at 3 mi (5 km), 5970 ft (1820 m). This is the lowest point on the Heather trail. The ten tent platforms are near the trail but well separated from each other. There's a creeklet immediately south. From here on, the path is trail width.

Five minutes past Buckhorn, look for orange tiger lilies in a depression. About ten minutes farther, a broad meadow grants a view of the the North Cascades spanning the southern horizon. Visible directly south is 8306-ft (2532-m) Castle Peak in Washington's Pasayten Wilderness.

From 4 mi (6.4 km) on, the trail winds through gently rolling subalpine meadows and among stands of coniferous trees. En route are seeps harboring elephant's head and white bog-orchids.

The stem and flowers of the elephant's head are pink-purple to reddish. The head and trunk of the elephant are only fingernail size. There are 6 to 12 rows of heads around the terminal end of the 8- to 15-inch (20- to 38-cm) stem. The bog orchid resembles a nun's hat. It has 10 to 30 tiny flowers on a green stem up to 25 inches (63 cm) tall.

At 5 mi (8 km), 6610 ft (2015 m), the Bonnevier trail forks right (southeast). Continue straight (northwest). A few minutes farther, attain a panoramic view southwest. The sharp peaks of the Hozomeen Range are prominent. Behind them are other peaks in North Cascades National Park, including 8906-ft (2715-m) Mt. Redoubt. Nearby south-southwest is twin-peaked, 7949-ft (2423-m) Frosty Mtn. Snow-capped 6726-ft (2050-m) Silvertip Mtn is northwest.

After passing 7031-ft (2143-m) **Big Buck Mtn**, enter a slabby depression where spreading phlox (white to pink) and penstemon (pink or purple) flourish. Visible ahead is 7452-ft (2272-m) First Brother Mtn. To the east are the low, forested mountains of the Interior Plateau.

Descend to reach a fork at 6.2 mi (10 km), 6824 ft (2080 m). The main trail proceeds northwest. Right leads 0.6 mi (1 km) generally north to 7454-ft (2272-m) **First Brother Mtn**. Atop the summit, looking south, you can see your starting point: Blackwall Peak. Second Brother Mtn is west. Third Brother Mtn is northwest.

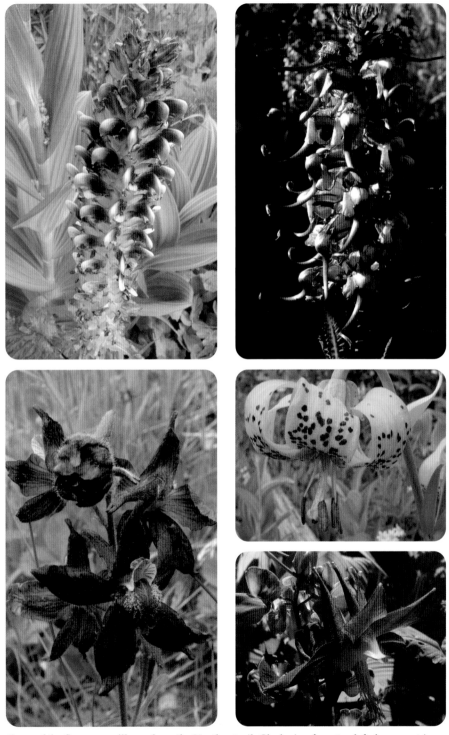

Some of the flowers you'll see along the Heather trail. Clockwise, from top left: lousewort in front of Indian hellebore, elephant's head, tiger lily, red columbine, larkspur.

Turning back at First Brother junction? Fast hikers can reach Buckhorn camp in one hour, the trailhead in two hours.

Proceeding northwest beyond First Brother, the trail skirts **Second and Third Brothers mountains**, both of which are slightly lower. In a basin between them is a reliable creek at 7.2 mi (11.6 km).

Low-growing plants are prevalent in the alpine tundra. One of them—moss campion—adapts to the short growing season and harsh conditions by spending nearly a decade nurturing a long tap root, by which it anchors itself and establishes a water supply. Only then do its tiny pink flowers blossom.

From the saddle below Third Brother, the trail descends 490 ft (150 m) into a basin. Reach **Kicking Horse camp** at 8.4 mi (13.5 km). Eight tent platforms are well off the trail to the left. Some have views of Third Brother. A creeklet crosses the main trail 0.3 mi (0.5 km) east of camp.

At 9 mi (14.5 km) the trail begins climbing out of Kicking Horse basin through rolling subalpine meadows. At 11.2 mi (18 km) drop 246 ft (75 m) into a forested bowl only to regain that elevation ascending the other side.

Pass two tarns at 11.7 mi (18.8 km). The trail levels, becoming narrow and less distinct. Continuing in subalpine forest, pass a third and fourth tarn. Right, slightly off the trail, is a view east across the Copper Creek drainage, toward Cathedral Lakes Provincial Park. Top out on **Nicomen Ridge** at 13 mi (21 km), 6562 ft (2000 m).

The view north makes it very apparent: you've hit the end of the North Cascades. Low, rolling, forested mountains spread north and east. If you're turning around here, first follow the trail far enough down the north end of the ridge to glimpse **Nicomen Lake** (northwest). The lakeside campground is at 14.3 mi (23.1 km), 5905 ft (1800 m).

From Nicomen Lake, it's possible to continue descending west 7 mi (11.5 km) on the Grainger Creek trail to a junction with the Hope Pass trail at 3199 ft (975 m), where left (southwest, paralleling the Skaist River) leads 5 mi (8 km) to **Hwy 3** at Cayuse Flats. Total one-way distance: 26.3 mi (42.3 km). But hitchhiking the 15.5 mi (25 km) back to Manning Park Lodge would be difficult. And you'd need a magic thumb to catch a ride from there, up the Cascade Lookout road, to the Blackwall Peak trailhead. A pre-arranged shuttle makes the one-way hike feasible, of course, but still not worthwhile. From Nicomen Lake to Hwy 3, the trail is entirely below treeline. Better to return the way you came, through the scenic meadows.

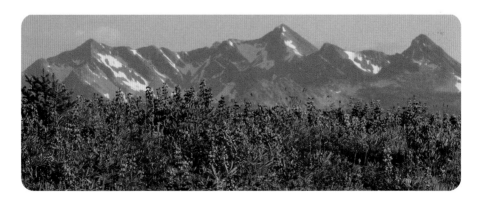

CATHEDRAL PROVINCIAL PARK

OPINION

Despite proof that the earth is round, apparently we kept wishing it were flat. Because we've succeeded in pounding much of our world flat again.

You now spend your life staring at flat surfaces: the pages of books, magazines, newspapers, computer screens, TV screens, movie screens. Even your car windshield creates the impression of watching a film.

And all this one-dimensional imagery, though mentally stimulating, requires you to be motionless, with your eyes focused on a fixed distance.

But you're a creature designed to move. So here's a trip that will keep you moving as nature intended—light, fast, and far—with only a daypack on your back, for three full days.

Cathedral Provincial Park in south-central British Columbia is the North Cascades' supreme basecamp/dayhiking destination. You'd have to travel to the Canadian Rockies to find anyplace comparable.

Above sweeping forested slopes, hidden from the valleys below, Cathedral is a high, lake-splashed, meadow-carpeted plateau with muscular topography. An exemplary trail network sleuths out all the optimal views of the surprisingly varied scenery and affords sustained alpine-zone hiking.

The 80,000-acre (33,000-hectare) park is distinct in the North Cascades, because it's at the outer limits of the range: north and east of Washington's rain forests, just shy of the arid Okanagan Highland farther north in British Columbia.

It's also distinct because it offers you a choice of accommodation. You can pitch your tent in a front-country-quality, lakeside campground. Or you can opt for a soft bed, hot shower and lavish meals in a lakeside lodge.

Before you make that choice, however, you must decide how to get there.

STORMING THE BASTILLE

Three trails—Lakeview Creek, Ewart Creek, Wall Creek—climb to the heart of Cathedral Park. All are trudgemills: long and steep. None is scenic. They're strictly utilitarian.

Your goal: dispatch the approach ASAP, so you can devote maximal time to the alplands above. So forget the Ewart and Wall creek trails. The Lakeview Creek trail—climbing 3848 ft (1173 m) in 10 mi (16.1 km)—is the most efficient access if you insist on hiking up, but under the burden of a full backpack, even it demands a day's slog.

Luckily, you have a fourth option. The lodge maintains a private 4WD road and several robust vehicles, so it can transport guests up and back. For a fee, non guests are welcome to ride too. Do it. You won't regret it.

What you will regret is wasting two full days should you hike up and back. We made that mistake once. Next time, we rode up in 45 minutes and spent the entire first day striding above treeline. We enjoyed another high-elevation hike the day we left. Riding down, we laughed at how stupid we'd been the first time.

Plan your trip to allow at least three days on top. That means you'll need five days if you hike up and back. That means you'll need a week if driving here from, let's say Seattle. Better to stay at the coal mine two extra days and use a portion of your earnings to pay for the lodge shuttle, and maybe even a room at the lodge.

NYLON OR SHINGLES

The Cathedral core-area campgrounds are excellent and in beautiful settings. Establish your dayhiking launchpad at Quiniscoe Lake, Lake of the Woods, or Pyramid Lake. (See photo on page 47.)

Quiniscoe is near the lodge and the road, plus the ranger cabin is located there, so it's the most convenient and popular. The other campgrounds feel wilder yet are only a 10- to 15-minute walk from Quiniscoe. Pyramid is the most scenic, with a fine view of its namesake mountain. Lake of the Woods has the most remote atmosphere.

Riding the lodge shuttle will enhance your camping experience by allowing you to pamper yourself with luxury camping gear you'd never wag on a back-pack trip: plush mattresses, pillows, chairs, a more spacious tent, camp shoes, a two-burner stove, and superior food. But bring your backpack anyway, to haul everything to your tentsite. You'll likely need a duffel bag too, to carry your daypack and whatever else doesn't fit in your backpack.

The option of cush camping might dissuade you from considering the lodge. But bear in mind, Cathedral Lakes Lodge is neither lavish nor preten-tious. It's comfortable, run by hikers for hikers. And their meals are delectable.

We've camped at Cathedral, and we've stayed in the lodge. We enjoyed both. You can pitch your tent throughout the North Cascades, however. This is the only remote lodge in the range and as such presents a unique opportu-nity. For a hiking-holiday splurge or a one-night indulgence, we enthusiasti-cally recommend it.

If we could, we'd return to Cathedral every summer, and we'd stay in the lodge. Learn more about Cathedral Lakes Lodge by visiting www.cathedral-lakes-lodge.com, or phoning 1-888-255-4453.

72-HOUR MINIMUM

The snowpack in Cathedral Park might curtail your hiking options until mid-July. In midsummer you'll see the wildflowers, but you'll share the trails with more hikers. The larches turn gold by mid-September.

Eager, athletic hikers who ride the lodge shuttle into and out of the park can explore most of Cathedral in a three-day blitz. Here's the optimal itinerary:

DAY ONE

Catch the first shuttle up. Hike to the Rim via Glacier Lake, continue to Stone City and Smokey the Bear, then return via Ladyslipper Lake.

DAY TWO

Hike to Lakeview Mtn, proceed to The Boxcar, drop to Goat Lakes, then return to Quiniscoe Lake.

DAY THREE

Hike the Red Mtn loop. Start early, so you'll have five hours to do it before catching the last shuttle down.

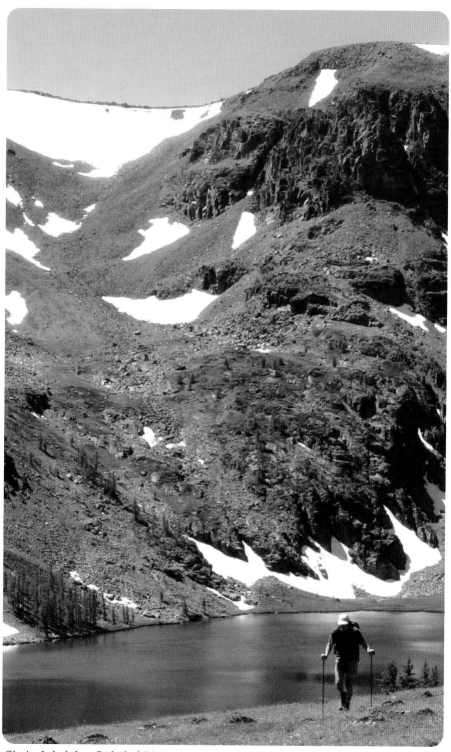

Glacier Lake below Cathedral Rim

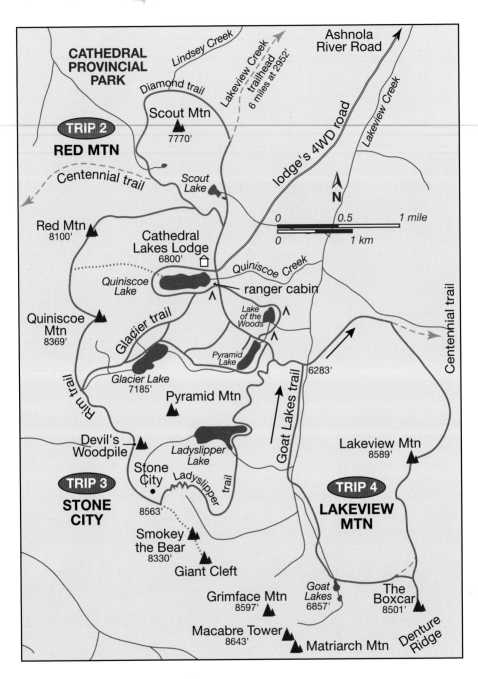

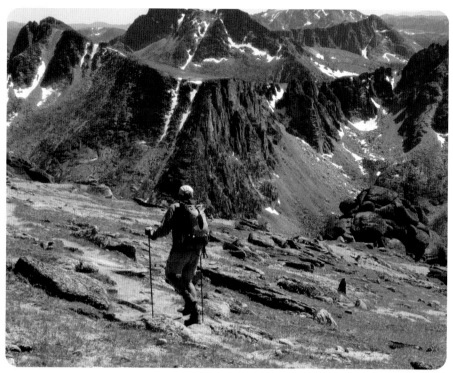

The rim trail, Cathedral Provincial Park

EYE ON THE SKY

The weather's good? Scurry onto the Cathedral Rim following directions for Stone City (Trip 3). This spectacular, high-elevation loop is your top-priority dayhike here. The Lakeview Mtn circuit (Trip 4) should be second on your list. The Red Mtn loop (Trip 2) should be third.

While on the rim, if you see serious weather approaching, get down quickly. You'd be a red flag for a bullish lightning bolt whether you're at the north end (8369 ft / 2551 m) or the south (8563 ft / 2610 m).

Even low clouds pose a threat on the rim. They can obscure the route and prevent you from following the cairns. The trails ascending to and descending off the rim are more rugged than maps indicate, so don't expect to clock your fastest-ever speeds here. But study a map anyway, so you'll know where your bailout options are.

If threatening weather keeps you off the rim, descend past Pyramid Lake to Lakeview Creek and Goat Lakes. If you're lucky, a break in the clouds will grant you a view of Denture Ridge taking a bite out of the sky. They should have named it Monster Mouth.

Glacier Lake is our favorite in Cathedral Park. Surrounded by mountains on three sides, it's a North Cascades alpine classic. You'll see it en route to Stone City (Trip 3) and again after traversing Red Mtn (Trip 2). But in sub-perfect weather, following the Trip 3 directions only as far as Glacier Lake is a reasonable option—short, not too high, but still scenic. Clouds permitting, you'll also see Lakeview Mtn (southeast) and the Similkameen Valley (northeast).

FACT

TRAIL NETWORK

The Cathedral Park trail network, radiating out from Quiniscoe Lake, is skookum. The tread is well maintained. Signs are neither in-your-face nor glaringly absent. And the entire network is accurately represented on the park map.

Some of the trails, however, are actually routes. Hiking across Lakeview Mtn to The Boxcar, for example, you'll be following cairns only. The rim-access routes are also not PCT quality, because the rough terrain they traverse doesn't allow it. But moderately experienced hikers should find them adequate and safe. In a whiteout, however, trying to follow these routes would be challenging.

The Stone City loop (Trip 3), the Lakeview Mtn circuit (Trip 4), and the Red Mtn loop (Trip 2) are, in that order, the premier dayhikes in Cathedral Park. Shorter dayhikes are also possible. Here are a few options, along with their approximate distance and elevation gain starting at Quiniscoe Lake:

Lake of the Woods / 0.8 mi (1.3 km) one way / level
Glacier Lake / 0.9 mi (1.5 km) one way / 410 ft (125 m)
Ladyslipper Lake / 1.9 mi (3 km) one way / 490 ft (150 m)
Goat Lakes / 3.1 mi (5 km) one way / 490 ft (150 m)

FLORA AND FAUNA

The Cathedral Park forests are predominantly Douglas fir at lower elevations, lodgepole pine a bit higher, Engelmann spruce and subalpine fir above, and Lyall's larch in the upper subalpine zone.

Botanists and birders visit the park every summer to observe more than 36 species of birds and scrutinize more than 500 varieties of plant life. The park harbors four of the North Cascades' eleven endangered plants. The ubiquitous wildflowers here are lupine, paintbrush, penstemon, and cinquefoil.

Is this grizzly-bear country? No. The resident griz population was exterminated long ago by ranchers. There are black bears in the park, but they tend to stay in the valleys, well below the park's core area, because it's such paltry dining for them above.

Cougar, mountain goats, bighorn sheep, wolverine, and mule deer inhabit the park. So do marmots and pika, which you might see on rocky outcrops in the alpine zone.

FISHING

Four of the Cathedral Park lakes were stocked with cutthroat and rainbow trout in the 1930s. Today, natural spawning maintains a healthy fish population. Pan-sized cutthroat are abundant in Lake of the Woods and Pyramid Lake. Trophy-sized rainbows lurk in Ladyslipper Lake.

BEFORE YOUR TRIP

Visit www.bcparks.ca to download the B.C. Parks map of Cathedral Provincial Park free of charge.

Be aware that mountain bikes are prohibited in the park. Dogs are forbidden around Quiniscoe Lake, to prevent them from harassing people and wildlife.

Make reservations with Cathedral Lakes Lodge for the 4WD shuttle on their private access road to Quiniscoe Lake in the park's core area. After checking the schedule and prices (www.cathedral-lakes-lodge.com) phone 1-888-255-4453.

From Keremeos in south-central B.C., drive Hwy 3 west. In 3 mi (4.8 km), turn left (south) onto the Ashnola River Road, cross the red bridge spanning the Similkameen River, and set your trip odometer to zero. Pavement ends at 6 mi (10 km).

You'll pass Ministry of Tourism campgrounds beside the Ashnola River at 7.6 mi (12.2 km), 8.5 mi (13.6 km), and 9.2 mi (14.8 km). Ignore the Ewart Creek bridge on the left at 9.6 mi (15.5 km). You're now in Cathedral Provincial Park. Pass an info kiosk on the right at 11.5 mi (18.5 km).

At 13.4 mi (21.5 km) reach the Cathedral Lakes Lodge parking lot. It's left, across the bridge. Their private 4WD road begins there and climbs to the lodge at Quiniscoe Lake.

If you're backpacking into the park, ignore the lodge parking lot. Continue driving the Ashnola River Road to 14.4 mi (23.2 km) and turn left at the sign for Lakeview Creek trailhead. Descend a rough 0.4 mi (0.6 km) to the road's end trailhead and campground at 2953 ft (900 m).

BC Parks allows backpackers to park here during their Cathedral trek and camp here the nights before and after, at no charge. The walk-in tentsites are 20 yd/m beyond the parking lot, near the Ashnola River, just downstream from the footbridge. There's an outhouse here but no tables. Fires are prohibited.

If you're backpacking into the park, your trek begins in the Lakeview Creek trailhead parking lot, at 2953 ft (900 m). Cross the footbridge over the Ashnola River, then ascend the trail southeast 0.6 mi (1 km) to the lodge's 4WD road.

Ascend the road, following the east bank of Lakeview Creek—locally referred to as Noisy Creek. At 1 mi (1.6 km), cross a bridge to the west bank.

At 2.2 mi (3.5 km) turn right, off the road, onto the signed trail. About halfway up, it's possible to pitch a tent near the north bank of Lindsey Creek. Farther southwest the trail breaks out of the trees and reaches a junction at 7.7 mi (12.4 km). Proceed straight (southwest) to reach Cathedral Lakes Lodge beside Quiniscoe Lake at 10 mi (16.1 km), 6800 ft (2073 m). Follow the trail around the lake's east end to reach Quiniscoe Lake campground.

There's a provincial-park ranger cabin above the southeast shore. Check in here, pay the camping fee, and get the park brochure/map. The tentsites are above the south shore of Quiniscoe Lake. Two more campgrounds are farther southeast, at Lake of the Woods and Pyramid Lake.

TRIP 2
RED MOUNTAIN

LOCATION	Cathedral Provincial Park, British Columbia
LOOP	8.1 mi (13 km)
ELEVATION GAIN	1640 ft (500 m)
KEY ELEVATIONS	trailhead 6759 ft (2060 m), Red Mtn 8100 ft (2469 m)
	Quiniscoe Mtn 8369 ft (2551 m)
HIKING TIME	4 to 6 hours
DIFFICULTY	moderate
MAPS	Cathedral Provincial Park (free download, www.bcparks.ca)
	Ashnola River 92 H/1 (Canada National Topo Series)

OPINION

Starting at Quiniscoe Lake, in the heart of Cathedral Park, three markedly different hiking experiences await, depending on which way you point your boots.

In this direction, you'll find the terrain less taxing, more pastoral. The trail swings around Scout Mtn, whose meadowy slopes have high-caliber flower power. Among the area's most visually strident blossoms are fleabane, lupine, cinquefoil, and yellow aster.

Like Cathedral's other two premier hikes, however, this one also leads above timberline, but less abruptly. After orbiting Scout Mtn, you'll rise onto the northern reaches of the Cathedral Rim, summitting first Red Mtn, then Quiniscoe Mtn, before plummeting to Glacier Lake.

Strong winds often pummel Cathedral Park, which means you should expect to be pummelled yourself, or at least roughed-up a bit, while hiking the rim. It's actually a blessing, because it keeps mosquitoes and flies clinging and cowering below rather than bedevilling you.

True to its name, Red Mtn is a pile of chunky, rouge-coloured boulders— a vivid contrast from Stone City, farther south on the rim, where the granitic gravel underfoot is virtually achromatic.

Atop Red and Quiniscoe mountains, you can proclaim yourself the benevolent monarch of all you survey. And you'll survey a lot: from the Thompson Plateau and Okanagan Highland farther north in British Columbia, to the rest of the North Cascades looming just across the border in Washington.

Atop Quiniscoe, your view of Cathedral Lakes basin improves. Four of the area's five primary lakes are visible: Quiniscoe, Glacier, Pyramid, and Lake of the Woods. Only Ladyslipper remains hidden.

The Glacier Lake cirque wins the Cathedral-pageant tiara, and you'll walk through it on the final leg of this trip. If you saw it previously while hiking the Stone City loop, all the better. Knowing what to expect, you'll feel even greater anticipation.

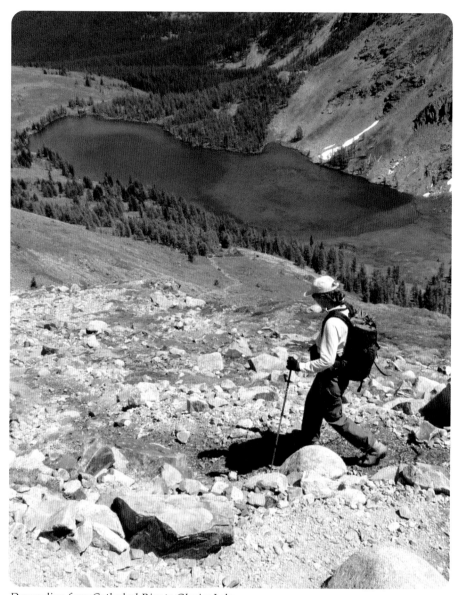

Descending from Cathedral Rim to Glacier Lake

FACT

See *Before your trip* and *By Vehicle* in the introduction to Cathedral Provincial Park on pages 42 and 43.

The following distances and times are based on starting at the BC Parks info kiosk near the Quiniscoe Lake outlet stream, at 6759 ft (2060 m). It's at the lake's east end, between Cathedral Lakes Lodge (above the northeast shore) and the campground and ranger cabin (above the southeast shore).

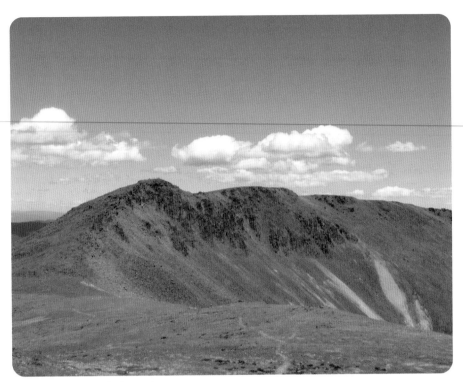

Gentle slopes on Red Mountain

ON FOOT

Walk toward the **lodge**, then proceed northeast on the road. It curves left and ascends. In one minute, fork right (northeast) onto the path signed for Scout Lake and the Diamond trail.

In 25 minutes, reach a junction at 0.5 mi (0.8 km), 6923 ft (2110 m). Left (northwest) ascends to Cathedral Rim and the Centennial trail. Continue straight (north). Three minutes farther, a spur forks left (northwest) to shallow **Scout Lake**. Proceed right (north) across a bridged stream.

About 45 minutes from the lodge, hike through a meadow ringed by pine and spruce trees. Fleabane, lupine, cinquefoil, and aster are abundant here. Five minutes farther, reach a junction at 1.6 mi (2.6 km), 7185 ft (2190 m). Turn left (northwest) onto the **Diamond trail** and begin a gentle ascent. Straight (north-northeast) is the Lakeview Creek trail, which descends all the way to the Ashnola River Road.

Rounding the north slope of **Scout Mtn**, the trail plies leafy meadows, returns to forest, then alternates between stands of trees and rocky clearings. The rolling, forested Thompson Plateau is occasionally visible northwest. Soon re-enter meadows.

Contour south, along the west slope of Scout Mtn, beneath the rounded, rock-strewn summit. Far northwest, Brothers Ridge is visible in Manning Park. Reach a junction at 3 mi (5 km), 7464 ft (2275 m), near a stand of larch. Right (west) is the **Centennial trail**, which descends, curving around the north and west slopes of Red Mtn. Go left (southeast) and ascend, following cairns up the grassy, rocky slope.

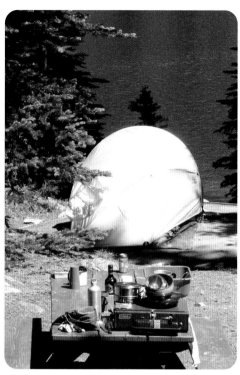

Quiniscoe Lake campsite

Lakeview Mtn is soon visible southeast. A bit farther, veer left, off trail, to overlook Scout Lake (northeast) in the basin below. At 3.7 mi (6 km), 7562 ft (2305 m) reach a junction with the rim trail. Straight descends southeast back to Quiniscoe Lake via the Scout Lake trail. Turn right and begin a gentle ascent west toward Red Mtn.

Denture Ridge, at the head of Lakeview Creek basin, is visible south-southeast. Lake of the Woods and Quiniscoe Lake are also now in view. Above Quiniscoe Lake is the east-jutting ridge of Quiniscoe Mtn. Behind that is Pyramid Mtn.

Follow cairns through chunky boulders to reach the first summit of **Red Mtn** at 4.5 mi (7.3 km), 8100 ft (2469 m). Five minutes farther, after a shallow dip, reach the second summit, where the bulk of the North Cascades is visible spanning the southwest horizon.

Following cairns, descend southwest over big, awkward boulders. About seven minutes below, reach a **saddle** at 5 mi (8 km), 7850 ft (2393 m). Left descends east to Quiniscoe Lake. Bear right and proceed south atop the rim.

A moderate ascent on a narrow trail marked by huge cairns leads to the 8369-ft (2551-m) summit of **Quiniscoe Mtn** at 5.6 mi (9 km). Glacier Lake is below (southeast). Also visible are, from left to right, Quiniscoe Lake, Lake of the Woods, and Pyramid Lake.

Descend southwest, then curve south to reach a signed junction at 6.5 mi (10.5 km), 8031 ft (2448 m), ten minutes below the summit of Quiniscoe Mtn. The rim trail continues south to Stone City. Turn left and begin the steep, rugged descent northeast to Glacier Lake.

Near the southwest end of **Glacier Lake**, ignore a right fork descending to follow the northwest shore. Proceed straight (northeast), staying above the lake. A few minutes farther, ignore another right fork descending to Glacier Lake but signed for Pyramid Lake. Proceed straight (east-northeast).

After a steep-but-short descent northeast, intersect the trail circling Quiniscoe Lake. You're above the south shore. Left rounds the west shore. Turn right, enter the campground, and proceed through it. Soon pass in front of the ranger cabin.

About one hour after departing the rim, reach the BC Parks info kiosk at the east end of **Quiniscoe Lake**, near the outlet stream, at 8.1 mi (13 km), 6759 ft (2060 m).

TRIP 3
STONE CITY

LOCATION	Cathedral Provincial Park, British Columbia
LOOP	8.2 mi (13.2 km) including Cathedral Ridge foray
ELEVATION GAIN	2730 ft (832 m)
KEY ELEVATIONS	trailhead 6759 ft (2060 m), junction on rim near Stone City 8563 ft (2610 m), Ladyslipper Lake 7283 ft (2220 m)
HIKING TIME	5 to 7 hours
DIFFICULTY	moderate
MAPS	Cathedral Provincial Park (free download, www.bcparks.ca) Ashnola River 92 H/1 (Canada National Topo Series)

OPINION

Hiking the Stone City loop is the quintessential Cathedral Park experience. Plan to do it the day you'll most likely have optimal weather.

The trail immediately flings you into the alpine zone via Glacier Lake cirque—the first of several destination-quality sights on this trip. A lunch stop here would be de rigueur had you not left the trailhead a mere 25 minutes before.

Above the lake, you'll crest Cathedral Rim where, on a clear day, it's instantly apparent why getting up here is mission critical for Cathedral hikers. In addition to the Cathedral Lakes basin, out of which you just ascended, you'll see a huge swath of the mountains along the Pacific Crest: from the B.C. Coast Range to, believe it or not, Mt. Rainier—200 mi (322 km) distant, near Seattle. Of course Mt. Baker also figures prominently in that panorama.

Even if the shark's mouth horizon isn't entirely visible, simply walking the rim trail is an event in itself. How often in the North Cascades, or any other range, do you get to stride (not struggle) above 8000 ft (2438 m) for any significant distance? Here you'll do it for 3 mi (4.8 km) if you follow the complete directions below.

Eons ago, when glaciers were busy buffing the eccentricities out of much of the Cathedral area topography, they missed a few things. Like the wind-eroded quartz formations at Stone City, where mountain goats often hang out and patiently pose for photos.

Smokey the Bear is another of the glaciers' oversights. It's a sheer-sided promontory atop the rim. Squint at it, and you might see Smokey's image set in stone. Or not. But if you veer off trail and hike to the top, you can look straight down the rim's vertical northeast side—a much more impressive sight than a nebulous cartoon bear.

Beyond Smokey, the rim trail dwindles and descends steeply to the Giant Cleft—a startling breach in the rim that's worth seeing mostly because getting there is an engaging romp.

When it's time to bail off the rim, that too is exciting. You'll meander across steep talus, enjoying constant views until gliding through larch forest to

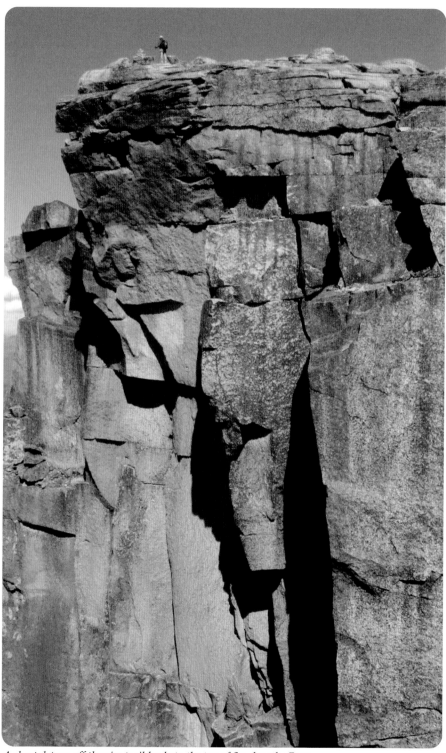

A short detour off the rim trail leads to the top of Smokey the Bear.

Ladyslipper Lake. If wind isn't ruffling the water, stop at the shore. Stare into the depths. You'll almost certainly see trout. Lots of 'em.

Only on the descent past Ladyslipper will you come down to earth, figuratively as well as literally. The trail is in forest the rest of the way, but the distance to your starting point is now short.

You'll see Pyramid Lake beneath its namesake peak—which you just finished circumambulating. And you can, if you have a bit more energy and curiosity, detour around Lake of the Woods for one final photo op before reaching Quiniscoe Lake.

FACT

See *Before your trip* and *By Vehicle* in the introduction to Cathedral Provincial Park on pages 42 and 43.

The following distances and times are based on starting at the BC Parks info kiosk near the Quiniscoe Lake outlet stream, at 6759 ft (2060 m). It's at the lake's east end, between Cathedral Lakes Lodge (above the northeast shore) and the campground and ranger cabin (above the southeast shore).

ON FOOT

Pass in front of the ranger cabin. Keep bearing right through the campground. In five minutes, go left (south) on the signed **Glacier trail**. Begin a steep ascent. The grade eases in larch forest. Lupine line the path.

Enter a level, alpine meadow at 7343 ft (2238 m), about 25 minutes from the trailhead. Ignore the left fork (signed for Pyramid Lake) descending southwest to **Glacier Lake**, which is visible below. Proceed straight (west-southwest), staying above the lake.

Near Glacier Lake's southwest end, ignore another left fork descending to follow the northwest shore. Proceed straight through a few trees, then begin a steep, switchbacking ascent generally southwest across loose rock. Purple penstemon and yellow cinquefoil adorn the dryas. Reach a T-junction atop **Cathedral Rim** at 1.6 mi (2.5 km), 8048 ft (2453 m), about an hour from the trailhead.

Right (north) ascends Quiniscoe Mtn and continues over Red Mtn. Go left (south) for Stone City. The bulk of the North Cascades are visible spanning the horizon: west to southwest.

At 2.2 mi (3.6 km) cross the **Devil's Woodpile**—a formation of columnar-jointed rocks apparently named by someone with a pathological fear of Satan. The trail continues south, dropping slightly then ascending on granite gravel.

At 2.7 mi (4.4 km), 8497 ft (2590 m), reach **Stone City**, a quartz monozonite formation untouched by the ice-age glaciers but eroded by wind. Mountain goats frequent the outcrops punctuating this moonscape.

A few minutes farther (east-southeast) reach a signed **junction** at 2.9 mi (4.7 km), 8563 ft (2610 m). Left (northeast) descends to Ladyslipper Lake. That's the way to continue looping back to Quiniscoe Lake. Right (south-southeast) is a spur probing Cathedral Ridge. A foray in that direction leads to Smokey the Bear and the Giant Cleft—a 1.6 mi (2.6 km) round trip.

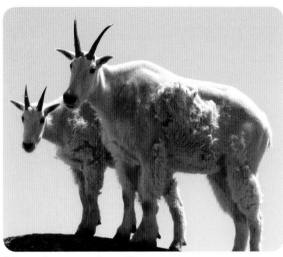

Mountain goats at Stone City

The cairned Cathedral Ridge spur descends, weaving through boulders. Within five minutes, pass a huge cleft. Ahead (southeast) is Grimface Mtn. Far south, Redoubt Mtn and even Glacier Peak are visible in Washington.

At 3.5 mi (5.6 km), 8317 ft (2535 m) reach a sign pointing to **Smokey the Bear**. It's the sheer promontory left (east). Supposedly the formation's silhouette resembles the famous bear. Ascending it, however, is more fun than puzzling over its appearance. You can reach the cairn on top in a quick detour.

Continue following the Cathedral Ridge spur generally southeast. Descending sharply, the trail dwindles to a route but remains distinct. Follow it among boulders, down scree, and along ledges to 3.7 mi (6 km), 8097 ft (2468 m), where a sign points left (north) up a steep chute to the **Giant Cleft**. It formed when a vertical seam of softer basalt eroded, leaving a deep, narrow gap between granite walls.

From the Giant Cleft, retrace your steps generally northwest 0.8 mi (1.3 km) to the **junction** just shy of Stone City, where your total distance will be 4.5 mi (7.3 km). Resume the loop by turning right and descending northeast.

It's a steep route across talus, curving east then southeast. About 30 minutes below the rim, curve north into the subalpine zone. Enter larch forest. The grade eases, and you're again on a comfortable trail.

At 5.8 mi (9.3 km), 7283 ft (2220 m), about an hour after departing the rim, reach the the southeast shore of **Ladyslipper Lake**. Bear right, cross the bridged outlet stream, and follow the trail along the west shore.

From the lake's northeast shore, ascend over a 7480-ft (2280-m) shoulder. A long descent ensues, northeast then generally north.

At 7.2 mi (11.6 km), 6719 ft (2048 m), about 30 minutes from Ladyslipper Lake, intersect the **Centennial trail**. Bear left (west-northwest) for Quiniscoe Lake, which is about 30 minutes distant. Right leads to Goat Lakes and Lakeview Mtn.

Ignore the left spur to Pyramid Lake. Cross Pyramid Lake's bridged outlet stream. Ignore the right fork descending to Lake of the Woods. Ignore the left fork ascending to Glacier Lake. Enter the **Quiniscoe Lake campground**.

About two hours after departing the rim, reach the BC Parks info kiosk at the east end of **Quiniscoe Lake**, near the outlet stream, at 8.2 mi (13.2 km), 6759 ft (2060 m).

TRIP 4

LAKEVIEW MOUNTAIN / THE BOXCAR

LOCATION	Cathedral Provincial Park, British Columbia
CIRCUIT	10 mi (16.1 km) including The Boxcar
ELEVATION GAIN	3228 ft (984 m) including The Boxcar
KEY ELEVATIONS	trailhead 6759 ft (2060 m), lowpoint at Lakeview Creek 6283 ft (1915 m), Lakeview Mtn 8589 ft (2618 m) The Boxcar 8501 ft (2591 m), Goat Lakes 6857 ft (2090 m)
HIKING TIME	7 to 8 hours
DIFFICULTY	moderate
MAPS	Cathedral Provincial Park (free download, www.bcparks.ca); Ashnola River 92 H/1 (Canada National Topo Series)

OPINION

Of Cathedral Park's three premier dayhikes, this circuit is the loneliest. During midsummer, we encountered hikers throughout the park, but none here.

That's because the trail is longer and more arduous. It tops out higher than the others—on the 8589-ft (2618-m) summit of Lakeview Mtn—plus it descends to Lakeview Creek both going and coming. The resulting elevation gain is significantly greater than on the other hikes, which ascend without interruption.

The Boxcar also requires a smidge of scrambling—easy and unexposed, but scrambling nonetheless. And the Lakeview-to-Boxcar section is a route, not a trail. It traverses rocky, alpine terrain where the tread is scant. You'll need a couple molecules of navigational sense, but if you're a moderately experienced hiker you should find it more exhilarating than troubling.

All this extra effort is worth it, and not only for the solitude you'll likely find. Touring the eastern reaches of the park's core area, you'll explore a greater variety of terrain, and you'll enjoy the most comprehensive view of Cathedral Lakes basin.

The descent to Lakeview Creek is a mere dip compared to the screaming plunges so often required in the North Cascades. Thankfully, this is not one of the deep, dark "holes" characteristic of the range. It's a shallow, forested drainage, nothing more, so you'll bottom-out quickly.

On the ensuing climb, you'll soon enter the subalpine zone, where streamlets writhe through meadowy slopes, and paintbrush and lupine grow in hothouse profusion. The forest thins and views expand within 45 minutes. To a hiker, striding through alplands like these ranks right up there with food, shelter, clothing and sex. It's a basic necessity of life.

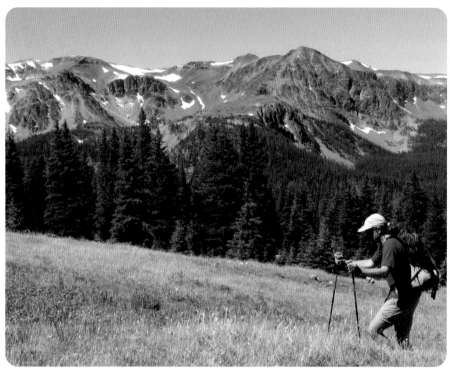

Ascending Lakeview Mountain, with Cathedral Rim across the valley

The growing panorama to the west is especially intriguing if you've already hiked the Cathedral Rim via Trips 2 and/or 3. It includes Ladyslipper, Glacier and Quiniscoe lakes, as well as the rim itself.

Atop Lakeview Mtn, the turbulent topography ringing Goat Lakes basin is impressively close: Denture Ridge, Matriarch Mtn, Macabre Tower, Grimface Mtn. Also visible are the Giant Cleft and Smokey the Bear.

On the clockwise circuit described below, you'll descend south off Lakeview Mtn into a saddle dividing it from The Boxcar. Don't let your momentum tempt you to blow off the Boxcar ascent and continue descending to Goat Lakes.

The Boxcar is a flat-topped butte with mini-summits at each end (east and west) that give it a vaguely boxcar shape. If you're imaginative, that is. And drunk. Scurrying up is fun. So is wandering on such a high, broad plain. You'll discover a queer contrast: sensuous granite above chaotically amorphous rock. You can peer into the surrounding valleys and scope-out the route to the distant Haystack Lakes.

Starting at Quiniscoe Lake, fit hikers can complete the Lakeview Mtn / Boxcar circuit in six hours. But if it's a warm, sunny day, and especially if it's calm, stay high as long as possible. Allow an additional hour for a skyline snooze. After descending into the larch forest below the Boxcar, you're unlikely to linger at the Goat Lakes. The setting is beautiful, but you'll have already seen the basin from above, atop the Boxcar's west summit.

FACT

See *Before your trip* and *By Vehicle* in the introduction to Cathedral Provincial Park on pages 42 and 43.

The following distances and times are based on starting at the BC Parks info kiosk near the Quiniscoe Lake outlet stream, at 6759 ft (2060 m). It's at the lake's east end, between Cathedral Lakes Lodge (above the northeast shore) and the campground and ranger cabin (above the southeast shore).

ON FOOT

Follow the trail south-southeast: the direction of Pyramid Lake. Left (northeast) leads to Lake of the Woods.

Ignore the right fork ascending to Glacier Lake. Ignore the left fork descending to Lake of the Woods. Cross Pyramid Lake's bridged outlet stream. Ignore the right fork to Pyramid Lake.

About 30 minutes from Quiniscoe Lake, reach a junction at 1 mi (1.6 km), 6719 ft (2048 m). Right (south-southwest) ascends to Ladyslipper Lake. Go left (southeast).

At 1.4 mi (2.3 km), 6398 ft (1950 m), about 40 minutes from Quiniscoe Lake, reach another junction. Right leads south-southeast to Goat Lakes. You'll return on that trail after completing the clockwise circuit described here. For now, go left (northeast), descending deeper into the fir-and-spruce forest.

About six minutes farther, at 6283 ft (1915 m), cross the bridge to the east bank of **Lakeview Creek**. Begin ascending northeast.

A steady, moderate-to-steep, half-hour ascent ensues. Enter the subalpine zone at 7087 ft (2160 m). Lupine dominate the pocket meadows. Creeklets cascade down the slope, dodging stands of alpine fir.

Still below the ridgecrest, reach a signed junction. Left (east-northeast) is the cairned Centennial trail, which continues to Twin Buttes and beyond. Go right (east-southeast) on a barely perceptible route across grass and granite scree, toward the blunt crest.

Boulders invite you to sit and appreciate the view you've earned. Matriarch Mtn is south-southwest. Right of it is Grimface Mtn. The clefts in Cathedral Ridge are southwest. Right of them is Stone City and the descent route above the Ladyslipper Lake cirque. Cathedral Rim is west. Scout Mtn is northwest, at the rim's north end. About ten minutes farther, Ladyslipper Lake is also visible.

At 3 mi (5 km), reach a 8268-ft (2520-m) saddle on the **ridgecrest**, where granite rocks are festooned with black lichen, and dwarf mountain-lupine is profuse. Follow the route south, curving southwest toward the summit.

At 3.7 mi (6 km), 8497 ft (2590 m), about 30 minutes above the Centennial-trail junction, the route passes immediately east of the 8589-ft (2618-m) summit of **Lakeview Mtn**. The complex summit ridge is strewn with granite slabs and chunky boulders, which were untouched by the glaciers that scoured Cathedral Park's lower elevations.

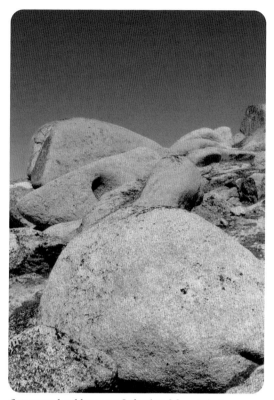

Sensuous boulders atop Lakeview Mountain

It takes only a few minutes to scamper up the summit, where Mt. Baker is visible west-southwest, 75 mi (120 km) distant. Nearby (south-southwest to southwest) are Denture Ridge, Matriarch Mtn, Grimface Mtn, and Macabre Tower. Behind them are the snowy peaks of Washington's North Cascades. South of and below the summit is a crude, stone windblock.

The cairned route descends south from the summit of Lakeview Mtn, gradually steepening. It wends through boulders to a **saddle** at 4.5 mi (7.3 km), 7940 ft (2420 m). To surmount The Boxcar, continue straight (south) and ascend the path bootbeaten into the scree. This out-and-back foray will add only about 1.5 mi (2.4 km) to your total distance.

About 20 minutes above the saddle, crest the 8379-ft (2554-m) midsection of **The Boxcar**. There are minor summits at each end of this generally level butte. Glacier Peak is now visible southwest, 80 mi (128 km) distant.

Go left (southeast) to the butte's 8501-ft (2591-m) east summit, where you can see the ridge route traversing Haystack Mtn to reach the Haystack Lakes, which are hidden from view. Then turn west and follow the butte's south edge. Double-Distilled Pass is visible below (west-southwest). Mountaineers descend off the pass to the Goat Lakes. Proceed to the butte's 8494-ft (2589-m) west summit to peer into the Goat Lakes basin.

After descending back to the **saddle** between The Boxcar and Lakeview Mtn, your total distance will be 6 mi (9.7 km). Turn left (west) and descend. Glissade through the scree, then pick up the obvious trail. About seven minutes below the saddle, enter larch forest at 7579 ft (2310 m).

About 17 minutes below the saddle, cross a reliable stream. Continue the descent to reach **Lakeview Creek** near where it flows from the **Goat Lakes**, at 6.7 mi (10.8 km), 6857 ft (2090 m). The area is swampy.

Go left (south) about 25 m/yd. Where the trail fades, proceed right (west) 40 m/yd. Regain the trail on the far side of the drainage, near the north lake—the larger of the two.

To complete the circuit, turn right and hike north-northwest through forest. The trail follows Lakeview Creek downstream. The creek is audible but not visible.

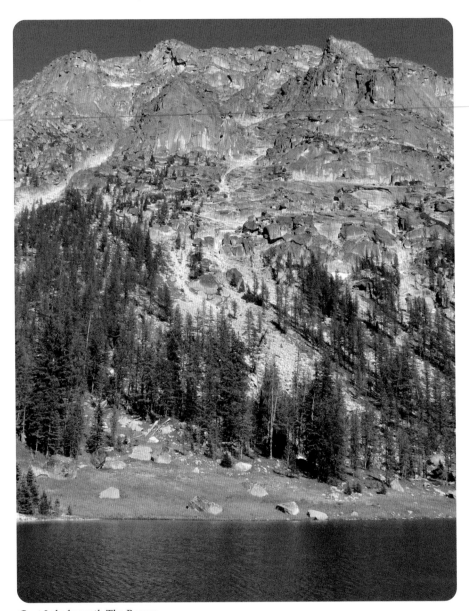

Goat Lake beneath The Boxcar

At 8.6 mi (13.8 km), 6398 ft (1950 m) intersect the **Centennial trail**. You're now on familiar ground. Right descends to cross Lakeview Creek. Turn left (northwest) and ascend. Your starting point is just 40 minutes away.

After passing between Pyramid Lake and Lake of the Woods, reach the BC Parks info kiosk at the east end of **Quiniscoe Lake**, near the outlet stream, at 10 mi (16.1 km), 6759 ft (2060 m).

TRIP 5
HELIOTROPE RIDGE

LOCATION	Mt. Baker Wilderness
ROUND TRIP	6.5 mi (10.5 km)
ELEVATION GAIN	1900 ft (580 m)
KEY ELEVATIONS	trailhead 3700 ft (1128 m), highpoint 5600 ft (1707 m)
HIKING TIME	4 to 6 hours
DIFFICULTY	moderate
MAP	*Green Trails* Mt. Baker 13

OPINION

It's amazing that with no skill whatsoever, without knowing how to do anything more complicated than walk, people can get to a place so other-worldly as this. Within a couple hours, you can be looking down on a living glacier from a vantage point high on a sleeping volcano. The hike is not only quick and easy, it's pleasant. The gentle ascent is through luxuriant forest cleaved by jubilant creeks.

At trail's end, the Coleman Glacier gnashes its way down the yawning abyss immediately below you. To the northeast is Chowder Ridge. Above, the summit of Mt. Baker is hidden behind its massive, gleaming white girth. Once

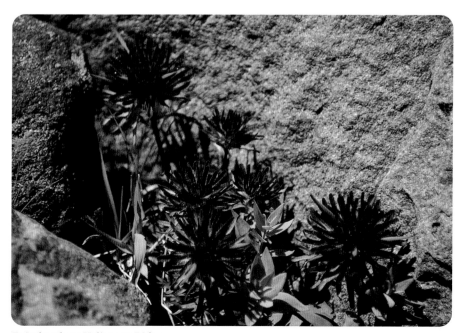

Paintbrush on Heliotrope Ridge

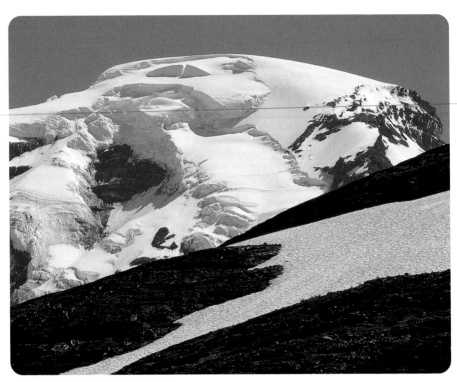

Mt. Baker, from Heliotrope Ridge

onto the moraine, you can explore. Or simply ponder existence. Just don't venture onto the ice without the knowledge and equipment to do it safely.

Though Heliotrope is tremendous, if you have to choose just one hike on Mt. Baker, and the incomparable Ptarmigan Ridge sounds too difficult for you or is still snow-covered, hike the nearby Skyline Divide. There, views of Mt. Baker glaciers are more expansive, green meadows add contrast to the scenery, clearcuts are not so readily visible, and you can roam longer at high elevation.

Some years, the Heliotrope trail is snow-covered until August, other years it's hikeable by early July. Check the Glacier Public Service Center before setting out. Even if you're told it's hikeable, carry trekking poles. They're always useful, and here they might prove invaluable on the unbridged stream crossings.

FACT

BY VEHICLE

From the Glacier Public Service Center, drive east on Hwy 542. At 0.8 mi (1.3 km), turn right onto Glacier Creek Road 39, reset your trip odometer to zero, and proceed south. Continue straight on the main road at 0.7 mi (1.2 km) and 7.8 mi (12.6 km). Reach the shopping-mall-size trailhead parking lot at 8.2 mi (13.2 km), 3700 ft (1128 m).

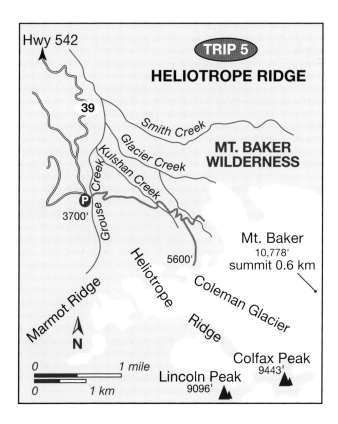

Hwy 542

TRIP 5
HELIOTROPE RIDGE

39

Smith Creek

Glacier Creek

Kulshan Creek

Grouse Creek

**MT. BAKER
WILDERNESS**

3700'

Mt. Baker
10,778'
summit 0.6 km

Heliotrope

5600'

Coleman Glacier

Marmot Ridge

Heliotrope Ridge

N

Colfax Peak
9443'

0   1 mile

Lincoln Peak
9096'

0   1 km

ON FOOT

The trail starts 30 yd/m left of the outhouse. It drops immediately into forest. Cross the bridge spanning deep, swift **Grouse Creek** and enter Mt. Baker Wilderness at 0.2 mi (0.3 km).

Begin a steep ascent generally east on a rocky, rooty, but serviceable trail. The grade relents near 0.5 mi (0.8 km). Views open to the north.

Beyond 1 mi (1.6 km) are several unbridged stream crossings. Earlier than mid-July, though the trail might be snow-free, high meltwater could make fording dangerous. The first stream, below a small waterfall, should pose no difficulty.

At 2 mi (3.2 km), between the first and second streams, pass a couple level, trailside tentsites. The second stream is in the subalpine zone: fewer trees, abundant heather, views to the icy realm above. The trail continues southeast.

Reach the third major stream at timberline. This one can be a more challenging ford; try to rockhop instead. Shortly beyond, reach the fourth major stream—actually several braided creeklets—at 2.4 mi (3.9 km). If you cross here, you'll follow a spur atop a small gravel ridge to a **Coleman Glacier overlook**.

To ascend as high as possible on Heliotrope Ridge, don't cross the fourth major stream. Opt for the bootbeaten climber's path ascending steeply right. It ends just above 5600 ft (1707 m) on a **moraine**, where a few hardy, red paintbrush and lavender sky pilot contrast vividly with the rocky rubble.

Given all day, it's easy to top-out high on Heliotrope Ridge *and* nip out to the Coleman Glacier overlook.

TRIP 6
SKYLINE DIVIDE

LOCATION	Mt. Baker-Snoqualmie National Forest
	Mt. Baker Wilderness
ROUND TRIP	10 mi (16.1 km) to saddle beneath Chowder Ridge
ELEVATION GAIN	2163 ft (659 m) to saddle
KEY ELEVATIONS	trailhead 4400 ft (1341 m), highpoint 6563 ft (2001 m)
	trail's end saddle 6300 ft (1920 m)
HIKING TIME	5 to 6 hours
DIFFICULTY	easy to moderate
MAP	*Green Trails* Mt. Baker 13

OPINION

There are many paths to Mt. Baker vistas. Some are long. Others are rigorous. This one's a shortcut—so easy it feels like you're cheating.

Just two miles of comfortable switchbacks deliver you to a sprawling meadow at the north end of Skyline Divide. From there on, it's an easy amble atop the crest, with the gleaming snowcone the centerpiece of an exploding panorama comprising peaks, valleys, waterfalls and tundra.

On a clear day, you'll see the Strait of Georgia and the mountains of Vancouver Island (west); British Columbia's Coast Range, the Border Peaks and the Cheam Range (north); and Mt. Shuksan (east). You'll also see Vancouver's billowing smog.

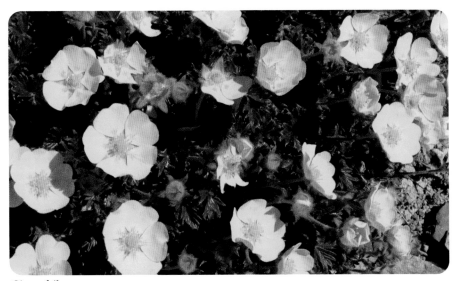

Cinquefoil

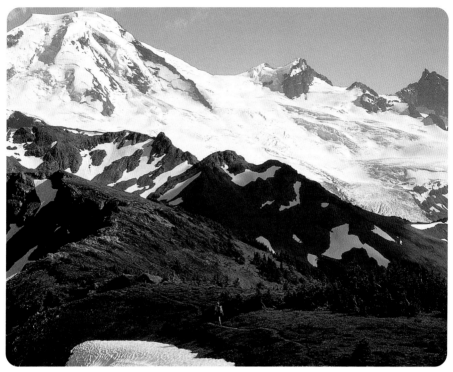

Skyline Divide, Mt. Baker

Despite the trail's popularity, it's possible to wander bluffs, basins and ridges away from the crowd. Solitude is more likely if you start hiking after 1 p.m. By the time you reach trail's end above Chowder Basin, the throng will have dispersed.

Solitude is guaranteed if you pitch your tent up there—on rock or dirt of course, never on tundra. With luck, a flaming sunset and rosy sunrise will enhance your view of Baker's lustrous glaciers.

Whether dayhiking or backpacking, carry all the water you'll need. Once the snow melts, you'll find no convenient source atop the divide.

You've been plagued by flies elsewhere in the North Cascades? You'll likely find them more tolerable here, even in August. And the resident butterfly population is booming. They will light on your hands and patiently pose for photographs.

FACT

BY VEHICLE

From the Glacier Public Service Center on Hwy 542, drive east 1 mi (0.6 km), turn right (south) onto Glacier Creek Road 39, and reset your trip odometer to zero. Immediately fork left onto Dead Horse Road 37. Proceed 4 mi (6.2 km) along the south bank of the North Fork Nooksack River. The next 8.9 mi (14.3 km) are rough and steep, climbing 2900 ft (884 m) via switchbacks. But a low-clearance 2WD car piloted by a patient driver can make it.

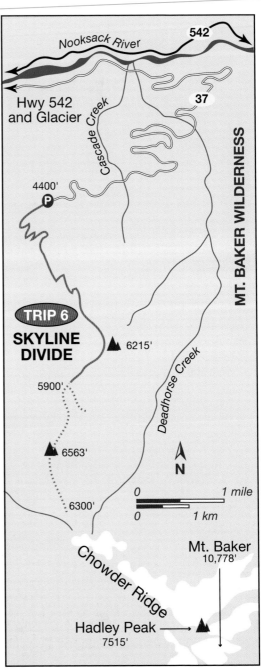
Reach the trailhead parking lot at 12.9 mi (20.8 km), 4400 ft (1341 m). The trail departs the upper end of the lot.

ON FOOT

After initially heading southwest, begin a switchbacking ascent southeast among hemlock and fir. Soon the forest is interspersed with meadows—flower filled in late July and early August.

After gaining 1400 ft (427 m) attain **Skyline Divide** at 2.25 mi (3.6 km), 5800 ft (1768 m). Proceed south. From here on, the trail follows the crest and is mostly above treeline.

At 2.75 mi (4.4 km) an obvious 6215-ft (1894-m) **knoll** just left (east) of the main trail affords a better view of Mt. Baker and allows you to survey the trail's southward progress.

Reach a fork at 3.5 mi (2.2 km), 5900 ft (1798 m). Left (southeast) drops to a water source and campsites in Chowder Basin, near the headwaters of Deadhorse Creek. Right undulates south, tops out at 6563 ft (2000 m), and ends at 5 mi (8 km) in a 6300-ft (1920-m) saddle near the base of **Chowder Ridge**.

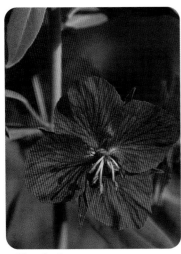

Willow-herb

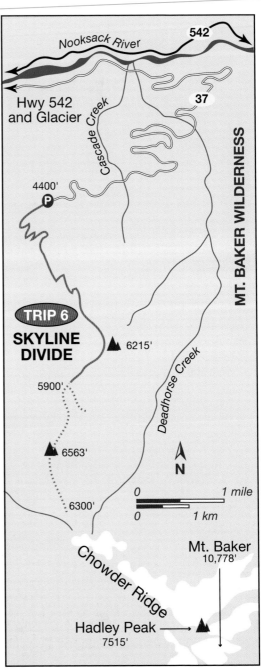

Nooksack River

542

37

Hwy 542 and Glacier

Cascade Creek

MT. BAKER WILDERNESS

4400'
P

TRIP 6

SKYLINE DIVIDE

6215'

5900'

Deadhorse Creek

6563'

N

6300'

0 ——— 1 mile
0 ——— 1 km

Mt. Baker
10,778'

Chowder Ridge

Hadley Peak ⟶
7515'

TRIP 7

EXCELSIOR RIDGE

LOCATION	Mt. Baker-Snoqualmie National Forest
ROUND TRIP	9 mi (14.5 km) to highpoint
ELEVATION GAIN	1780 ft (543 m)
KEY ELEVATIONS	trailhead 4150 ft (1265 m), Excelsior Pass 5350 ft (1630 m) highpoint 5930 ft (1808 ft)
HIKING TIME	4 to 5 hours
DIFFICULTY	easy
MAPS	*Green Trails* Mt. Baker 13, Mt. Shuksan 14

OPINION

Smell something burning? That would be your thighs, should you opt for one of the purgatorial ascent routes from Hwy 542 to Excelsior Ridge.

Hear something crackling? That would be your knee cartilege, should you opt to descend either of those triple-black-diamond slopes.

But suffering these abuses is unnecessary. Enjoying the spectacular views of Mt. Baker and Mt. Shuksan from Excelsior Ridge is easy. Simply drive to the Damfino Lakes trailhead, behind and just below the ridge.

Waddlers, toddlers, everyone finds comfort and joy on this gentle, merciful trail. The word *steep* does not apply here. Such a high-elevation start ensures the trees en route are too few to obscure views for long. Alpine blossoms are rife in summer. You'll enjoy big scenery nearly the whole way.

And if you're capable of those wicked ascent routes but wise enough to laugh them off, beginning your hike as described here will allow you to gallop cross-country through the alpine zone for a full day.

True, many hiker-accessible vantages boast views of Baker and Shuksan. What makes this one special is the High Divide trail linking Excelsior Pass with Welcome Pass. It traverses meadowlands on the south side of Excelsior

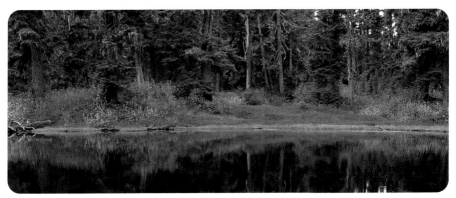

Damfino Lake

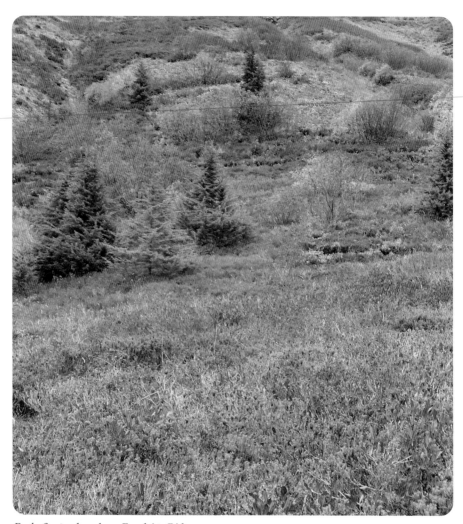

Early September along Excelsior Ridge

Ridge, directly across from the exalted mountains, separated from them only by the Nooksack River valley.

Once the trail is snow-free, usually in Late July, the optimal time to hike here depends on your color preference: bright green with a rainbow of wild-flowers in August, or yellows, golds, oranges, reds, and purples after mid-September. White—the color of the great glaciers draped across Baker and Shuksan—will be prevalent whenever you're here, as long as the sky is blue. If the weather forecast suggests it won't be, you'll miss the panorama that makes Excelsior Ridge a WOW destination.

Options: Less ambitious hikers aim for the humble summit of Excelsior Mountain, immediately above Excelsior Pass. Fit, eager striders turn around at the 4.5-mi (7.2-km), 5930-ft (1808-ft) highpoint beyond Excelsior Pass. Strong, adventurous explorers roam west of Excelsior Pass toward Church Mountain, or northeast of Welcome Pass to overlook the tarns in Yellow Aster basin

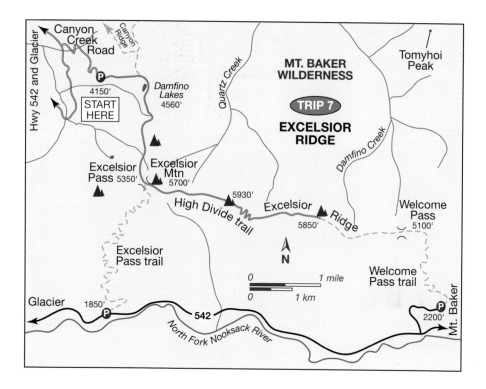

BY VEHICLE
From the Glacier Public Service Center on Highway 542, drive northeast and cross the bridge over the North Fork Nooksack River. At 1.8 mi (2.9 km) turn left (northwest) onto Canyon Creek Road 31, which loops from the west side of Church Mtn around to the northeast side of Bearpaw Mtn. Reset your trip odometer to zero. At 7 mi (11.3 km), pass Canyon Creek campground on the right. Pavement ends at 10 mi (16.1 km). At 14.6 mi (23.5 km) bear left (southeast) on Road 31. Reach the signed Damfino Lakes trailhead at 15.6 mi (25.1 km), 4150 ft (1265 m).

ON FOOT
The trail starts in the north corner of the parking lot, left of the sign. If you intend to camp, note that fires are prohibited within a mile of the trail. Ascend generally east into a regrowing clearcut.

In 15 minutes, reach a signed fork at 0.7 mile (1.1 km), 4600 ft (1402 m). Left (north-northwest) ascends past Cowap Peak to Canyon Ridge. Go right (east-southeast) and descend. Five minutes farther, pass the marshy **Damfino Lakes**, which are actually one contiguous pond.

Resume ascending generally south. About 40 minutes from the trailhead, reach a grassy bench at 5000 ft (1525 m). Proceed through a gap, into the alpine zone. Bearpaw Mtn is right (west). The meadows at 2.2 mi (3.5 km) are a flower garden in summer.

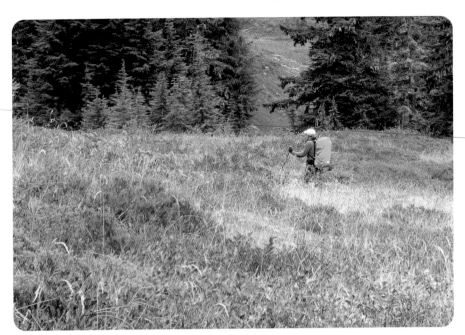

En route to Excelsior Pass

Reach a junction in **Excelsior Pass** at 3 mi (4.8 km), 5350 ft (1630 m). There are tentsites and a toilet here. Church Mtn is right (west). The right (southeast) fork descends 3500 ft (1067 m) in 4.2 mi (6.8 km) to intersect Hwy 542. Go left to continue on the **High Divide trail**, traversing east along the south slope of Excelsior Mtn toward Welcome Pass.

Just beyond the fork, bear right on the main trail where a left spur quickly ascends to the rounded, 5700-ft (1737-m) summit of Excelsior Mtn.

At 3.3 mi (5.3 km) enter Mt. Baker Wilderness. Ascend through heather and grass. Mt. Baker dominates the southern horizon. Crest the trail's 5930-ft (1808-m) **highpoint** at 4.5 mi (7.2 km).

Visible east-southeast, 9 mi (14.5 km) distant, is the Nooksack River canyon, a classic "deep hole"—the local term for the immense ravines that characterize the North Cascades. This one, beneath icy Mt. Shuksan, is 2000 ft (610 m) deep.

The trail proceeds east but descends nearly 500 ft (152 m) in 0.6 mi (1 km) before climbing back to 5460 ft (1664 m). Beyond, a virtually level mile precedes an ascent to 5850 ft (1783 m). Here, at 6 mi (10 km), Tomyhoi Peak is visible north-northeast.

Soon after, the trail descends again, reaching **Welcome Pass** at 7.5 mi (12.1 km), 5100 ft (1554 m). Then it drops into forest, curves right (south), and plunges 2400 ft (732 m) in 1.8 mi (3 km) via 67 switchbacks. The grade eases just before reaching Welcome Pass trailhead on Road 3060 at 10 mi (16.1 km), 2200 ft (671 m).

TRIP 8
CHURCH MOUNTAIN

LOCATION	Mt. Baker Wilderness
ROUND TRIP	8.4 mi (13.5 km)
ELEVATION GAIN	3600 ft (1097 m)
KEY ELEVATIONS	trailhead 2400 ft (732 m), highpoint 6000 ft (1830 m)
HIKING TIME	4 to 6 hours
DIFFICULTY	moderate
MAP	*Green Trails* Mt. Baker 13

OPINION

The tall, slender towers on a mosque are called *minarets*. Their needle-point shape was intended to pierce the sky, allowing the prayers of faithful Muslims to rise heavenward to Allah. Mountain devotees might attribute a similar spiritual purpose to the peaks they worshipfully hike and climb. If so, here's a fitting place to loft your reverent thoughts into the firmament: Church Mtn. It's in the heart of the North Cascades, with a nearly 360° panorama dominated by Mt. Baker.

But you'll work hard to reach this church. Come prepared with some deep thinking to do, plenty of stimulating questions to ask your hiking companion, or simply a need to meditate—anything to help pass the time on the steep, relentless switchbacks. There's little understory to make the forest more interesting, but at least there's no brush to tangle with. The roar of the Nooksack River in the valley below will accompany your heavy breathing on the ascent.

The wildflower-garden meadows cradled beneath the summit ridge are an idyllic place to relax before the final spurt to the top. Many hikers stop here with no intention of continuing. If you prefer to catch your breath in solitude, wander south toward the rim of the basin or proceed a quarter mile through the meadow.

Better yet, save your rest break for the top. The trail ends on the summit ridge, well shy of the climbers-only Church Mtn steeple, but the climactic vista is glorious. We saw a family—whose oldest child was ten and whose youngest was three—gleefully bounding up the final approach. So you probably can too, unless you're unnerved by the mild sense of exposure on the final 75 yd/m. Even if you go only a half mile beyond the creek crossing in the meadow, you'll earn a superior view.

The streams here are unreliable after July, so carry plenty of water. On a clear, hot day, you'll welcome the forest canopy on the taxing ascent. If the weather's threatening, go elsewhere. Poor visibility diminishes this hike to a mere training run. And the final approach is precariously slick when wet.

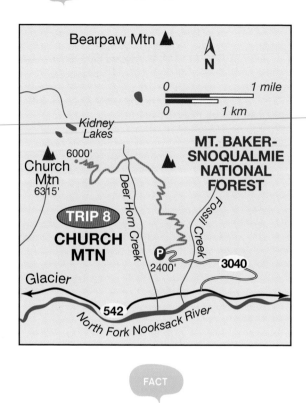

FACT

BY VEHICLE

From the Glacier Public Service Center on Hwy 542, drive 5.1 mi (8.2 km) east. Turn left onto Church Road 3040 and continue 2.6 mi (4.2 km) to the trailhead at 2400 ft (732 m).

ON FOOT

Follow a former logging road generally northeast 0.3 mi (0.5 km). Beyond an old clearcut at 0.8 mi (1.3 km), the trail is mostly in tall trees. Heading generally north-northwest, moderately-graded switchbacks steepen at 1.8 mi (2.9 km).

Near 2.2 mi (3.5 km), glimpse Mt. Baker (south). Pass a waterfall on the left at 2.5 mi (4 km). Soon after, the trail contours northwest into a basin. At 3.2 mi (5.1 km), 4900 ft (1494 m) enter a broad **meadow** tucked into the rugged slopes of Church Mtn. There's a seasonal creek here. Your goal—the summit ridge—is 1100 ft (335 m) above to the west.

At 3.5 mi (5.6 km) ascend open slopes festooned with corn lilies. The trail deteriorates at 4 mi (6.4 km) across a steep, bare, possibly muddy slope. Though the route is obvious, walking this short stretch is dicey in the rain. Reach **trail's end** at 4.2 mi (6.8 km), 6000 ft (1830 m). There's room for only about four people to safely, comfortably sit here. The craggy, 6315-ft (1925-m) summit of Church Mtn is nearby west-northwest.

If you've previously hiked Skyline Divide or Heliotrope Ridge on Mt. Baker, you'll find them easy to identify looking south from Church Mtn. On a clear day, Mt. Rainier is visible farther south. Mt. Sefrit and Icy Peak are east. Tomyhoi Peak and Mt. Larrabee are northeast. The Canadian Border Peaks are north. Below, to the north, are the Kidney Lakes. Clearcuts are visible in all directions.

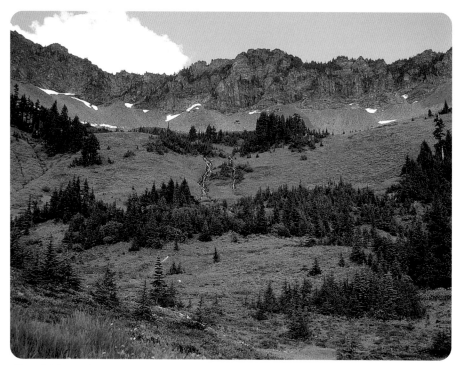

Church Mountain

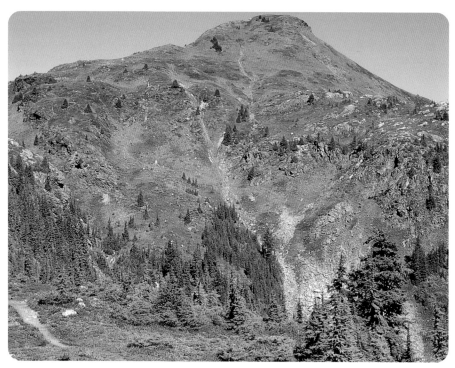

Yellow Aster Butte (Trip 9)

TRIP 9
YELLOW ASTER BUTTE

LOCATION	Mt. Baker Wilderness
ROUND TRIP	7 mi (11.3 km) to butte or tarns, 8 mi (12.9 km) to both
ELEVATION GAIN	2550 ft (777 m) to butte
KEY ELEVATIONS	trailhead 3600 ft (1098 m), butte 6150 ft (1875 m)
	tarns 5400 ft (1646 m)
HIKING TIME	4 to 5 hours
DIFFICULTY	moderate
MAP	*Green Trails* Mt. Shuksan 14

OPINION

Awesome as Mounts Baker and Shuksan are, after hiking several of the trails above Hwy 542 you might wonder: do any offer a different scenic climax? Yes, Yellow Aster Butte does. Although it affords yet another perspective of the lofty celebrities, you need never look in that direction to feel rewarded for your effort.

Hikers come here to revel in a vast undulating meadowland dimpled with a multiplicity of tarns. This is country made for wandering, not just picking a perch to eye the panorama. If you're not limited to a dayhike, pitch your tent—well off the trail, perhaps northeast or northwest of the tarns beyond the butte—and enjoy a second day of exploration. Ambling the alplands toward Tomyhoi Peak is a joy, though the final summit push is a technical climb.

By late July, the trail's namesake yellow asters (daisies) are abundant. In August, purple asters, pink and yellow monkeyflower, orange paintbrush, rosy spirea, and bistort light up the meadows. In fall, your hiking progress will likely be impeded by a bumper crop of berries—hucks and blubes.

Hikers are increasingly aware of their responsibility to leave no trace in the backcountry. But you'll see evidence that Yellow Aster Butte still attracts a few meadow-trampling morons. Do your best not to crush any more of the fragile, alpine greenery. If the tread is muddy, let your boots get muddy; sidestepping only broadens the mess. And certainly don't pitch your tent on grass. Opt for a bare tentsite where your impact will be minimal.

FACT

BY VEHICLE

From the Glacier Public Service Center on Hwy 542, drive east 12.8 mi (20.6 km). At the maintenance buildings, turn left (north) onto unpaved Twin Lakes Road 3065 and follow it 4.5 mi (7.2 km) to the trailhead parking on a tight switchback at 3600 ft (1098 m).

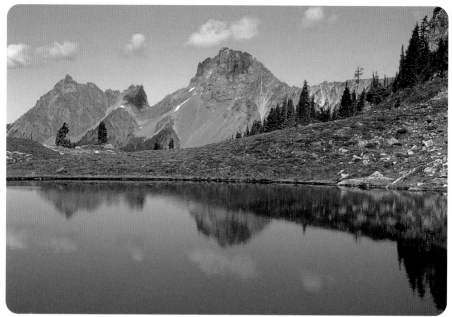

Tarn below Yellow Aster Butte, with American Border Peak in distance

ON FOOT

Ascend a well-constructed trail into beautiful, mature forest. The switch-backing ascent leads generally northwest.

After traversing left (west-southwest), curve north at 4560 ft (1400 m) into a meadowy basin. A cascade is visible above. Soon begin ascending again, past prolific berry bushes.

Reach a signed fork at 1.4 mi (2.3 km), 5200 ft (1585 m). Left (north-north-west) contours around the head of the basin and continues to Yellow Aster Butte. Right ascends north, cresting **Gold Run Pass** at 1.7 mi (2.7 km), 5500 ft (1676 m), en route to Tomyhoi Lake at 3.2 mi (5.1 km), 3700 ft (1128 m).

It's worth nipping up to the pass for a view. The pass itself is forested. Beyond, the trail plunges north-northeast. If you drop just 20 yd/m to the first switchback, Tomyhoi Lake is partially visible north-northwest.

After returning to the 1.4-mi (2.3-km) fork, proceed toward Yellow Aster Butte by contouring around the head of the basin: northwest, curving south-west. Twin-peaked Goat Mtn is visible left (southeast). Beyond it is Mt. Shuk-san. Mt. Baker is south-southwest.

After a bouldery stretch, the trail curves west then north again, revealing Tomyhoi Peak northwest beyond the tarns in Yellow Aster basin. At 3 mi (5 km), 5550 ft (1692 m) reach a junction: right ascends the butte, left descends to the tarns.

Turning right at the 3-mi (5-km) junction, begin the final, steep ascent generally north. Surmount the broad, flat, south end of **Yellow Aster Butte** at 3.5 mi (5.6 km), 6150 ft (1875 m). The mountainous panorama includes the wild Picket Range (southeast). A route continues north to the butte's marginally higher true summit.

Turning left at the 3-mi (4.8-km) junction, descend generally northwest to reach the **Yellow Aster tarns** in the basin west of the butte, at 3.5 mi (5.6 km),

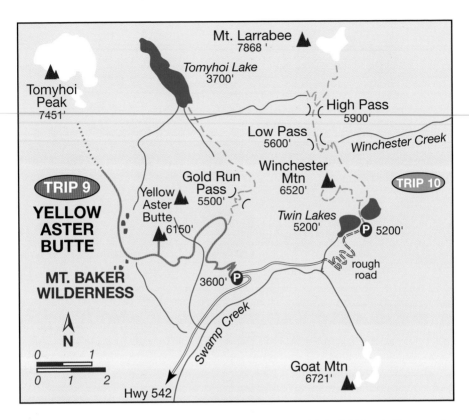

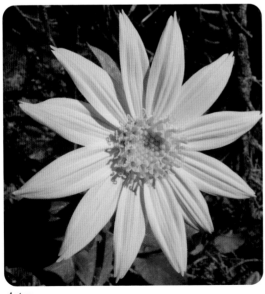

Aster

5400 ft (1646 m). Rusty mining junk litters the basin. Mt. Larrabee (northeast) and American Border Peak (north-northeast) are visible from the basin's north edge.

The route to 7451-ft (2271-m) **Tomyhoi Peak** will be obvious to anyone with cross-country experience. The peak's south ridge is surprisingly broad and gentle between 5800 ft (1768 m) and the 7000-ft (2134-m) false summit.

MT. LARRABEE

LOCATION	Mt. Baker Wilderness
ROUND TRIP	8 mi (12.9 km) to Winchester Mtn
	10 mi (16.1 km) to High Pass from Yellow Aster trailhead
ELEVATION GAIN	2920 ft (890 m) to Winchester Mtn
	2300 ft (701 m) to High Pass from Yellow Aster trailhead
KEY ELEVATIONS	Yellow Aster trailhead 3600 ft (1098 m)
	Twin Lakes trailhead 5200 ft (1585 m), Winchester Mtn
	6520 ft (1987 m), High Pass 5900 ft (1798 m)
HIKING TIME	4 to 6 hours
DIFFICULTY	moderate
MAP	*Green Trails* Mt. Shuksan 14

OPINION

Someday your life will flash before your eyes. Hiking in places like this will ensure your final flick is full of beautiful scenery. You'll behold Puget Sound, the British Columbia Coast Range, and many of the North Cascades' heavyweight mountains. Ideally, hike here in September, when the foliage is all sparks and fire. That way, when your body and soul part ways, you'll think you're exiting the world in a blaze of glory.

So, with two distinct destinations accessible from this trailhead, which should you aim for?

Winchester Mtn is a steeper climb, but the distance is shorter and there's a former fire-lookout cabin on the summit (which you can arrange to spend the night in) so it attracts a bigger crowd. The view is superb, comprising Mt. Baker, Mt. Shuksan, the Border Peaks, Silesia Creek valley, the jagged Pleiades beside Mt. Larrabee, and nearby Goat Mtn.

The view from High Pass, on the upper reaches of Mt. Larrabee, encompasses all that and more, including Artist Point (at the end of Hwy 542), Skyline Divide to the southwest, and Glacier Peak way south.

Winchester's only scenic advantage is a better view of the wickedly serrated Picket Range. Overall, High Pass affords a superior panorama, you'll likely share it with fewer hikers, plus the narrow tread and varied terrain en route give the journey a stronger whiff of wilderness.

So if you must limit yourself to just one of the two, make it High Pass. In a single day, however, strong hikers can easily tag High Pass, then zoom up and down Winchester on the way back. Plan on reaching both destinations, set out early for High Pass, then see if you have time and energy for Winchester. Another advantage of leaving Winchester 'til afternoon is that most hikers will have vacated the mountain before you begin ascending it.

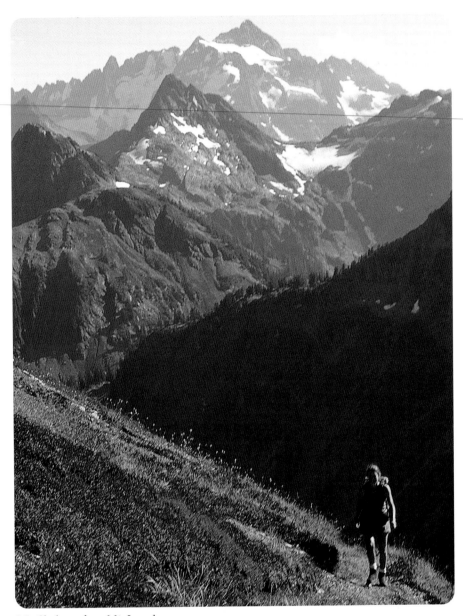

Mt. Shuksan, from Mt. Larrabee

FACT

BY VEHICLE

From the Glacier Public Service Center on Hwy 542, drive east 12.8 mi (20.6 km). At the maintenance buildings, turn left (north) onto unpaved Twin Lakes Road 3065 and follow it 4.5 mi (7.2 km) to the Yellow Aster Butte trailhead on a tight switchback at 3600 ft (1098 m).

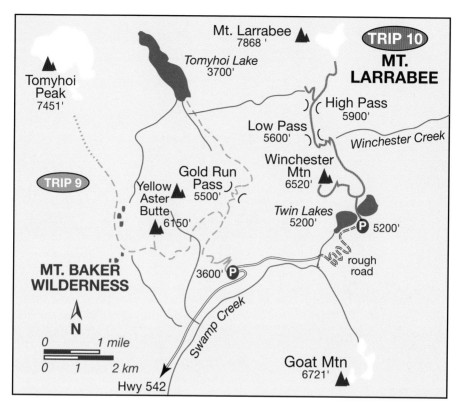

Mt. Larrabee ▲▲
7868 '

Tomyhoi Lake
3700'

TRIP 10

**MT.
LARRABEE**

▲
Tomyhoi
Peak
7451'

High Pass
5900'

Low Pass
5600'

Winchester Creek

Winchester
Mtn ▲
6520'

TRIP 9

Gold Run
Pass

Yellow ▲
Aster ▲
Butte
▲6150'

Twin Lakes
5200'

P 5200'

MT. BAKER
WILDERNESS

3600' **P**

rough
road

↑
N

Swamp Creek

0   1 mile

0   1   2 km

Hwy 542

Goat Mtn
6721'
▲▲

Any 2WD car can make it this far. The remaining 2.5 mi (4 km) are rough and narrow, steeply climbing 1600 ft (488 m) with dropoffs only a foot or less from your tires. The road crosses several ditches that might cause low-clearance cars to bottom out. In years of average or high snowfall, it probably won't be passable until mid-August, and even then will require 4WD and a capable driver. Ask the service center staff about road conditions. While you're at it, ask about trail conditions; hikers without ice axes might find snow patches obstructing safe passage until late August.

The road ends at 7 mi (11.3 km), 5200 ft (1585 m), near Twin Lakes. Most hikers park at the Yellow Aster trailhead and walk the final stretch of road.

ON FOOT

If you start at the Yellow Aster trailhead, add to your agenda a 5-mi (8-km) round-trip road walk during which you'll ascend and descend 1600 ft (488 m).

Upon arrival at the **road's end parking lot**, proceed to the trailhead on the northwest side of the isthmus between the Twin Lakes. Don't walk the gated road along the southeast side of the north lake.

Reach a fork in just 0.2 mi (0.3 km). Go left for Winchester, right for High Pass.

The switchbacking ascent to Winchester leads generally northwest among heather and a few trees. At 0.9 mi (1.5 km), the ascent eases, heading southwest. The final approach switchbacks generally north-northeast. Reach the 6520-ft (1987-m) **summit** at 1.5 mi (2.4 km). The former fire-lookout cabin here

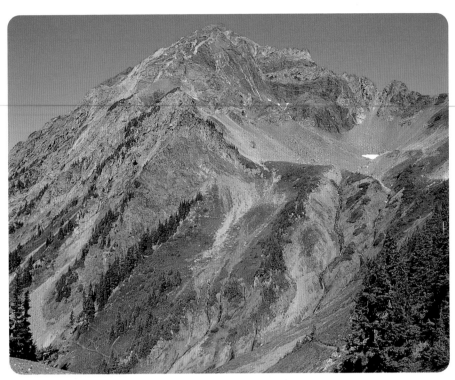

Mt. Larrabee, from Winchester Mountain

is open to the public July through September. For overnight reservations, contact the Mt. Baker Hiking Club: (360) 617-1219.

Heading generally north toward High Pass from the 0.2-mi (0.3-km) fork, quickly reach a small **saddle** affording a view of your goal—northwest, at the top of Mt. Larrabee's long south flank.

From the saddle, descend 160 ft (50 m), traversing under Winchester Mtn and proceeding northwest above the depths of Winchester and Silesia creek canyons. The trail then switchbacks up a rockslide to **Low Pass** at 1.5 mi (2.4 km), 5600 ft (1707 m). Continue generally north.

Reach 5900-ft (1798-m) **High Pass** at 2.5 mi (4 km). There's a fork here. Left descends to Gargett Mine at 5700 ft (1738 m). Right ascends higher on Mt. Larrabee, ending in about 1 mi (1.6 km) at 6500 ft (1982 m)—still well below the 7868-ft (2398-m) summit.

TRIP 11

GOAT MOUNTAIN

SHOULDER SEASON

LOCATION	Mt. Baker Wilderness
ROUND TRIP	8.4 mi (13.5 km)
ELEVATION GAIN	2950 ft (899 m)
KEY ELEVATIONS	trailhead 2500 ft (762 m), trail's end 5450 ft (1661 m)
HIKING TIME	3 to 4 hours
DIFFICULTY	moderate
MAP	*Green Trails* Mt. Shuksan 14

OPINION

In Washington, keen hikers ache most of the year. Not from hiking, but from the unfulfilled *desire* to hike. Snowdrifts that could bury an NBA team keep hiking season cruelly short in the North Cascades.

But there are a few places where, as early as May, snow is unlikely to impede your progress to a rewarding panorama. One of these trails ascends Goat Mtn, whose sun-blasted south-facing slope has on rare occasions been snow-free in April.

Shortly after setting out, you'll be looking across Nooksack River Valley at fearsome peaks that are thrillingly close. You'll even see Price Lake embedded in the shadows of Mt. Shuksan's steep walls, beneath Price Glacier. It's accessible only to satyrs—half man, half goat.

Shift your focus from macro to micro and you'll find Goat Mtn interesting from that perspective too. In season, glacier lilies, valerian, paintbrush, and tiger lilies grace the meadowed slopes. Images of luscious grass might linger in your mind long after hiking this verdant mountain reminiscent of the palis of Hawaii. Hear a whirring sound? Goat Mtn seems to be a hummingbird haven.

Obviously, the earlier you attempt Goat Mtn, the more likely you are to encounter snow and the lower it'll be. Before setting out, ask at the Glacier Public Service Center about trail conditions. Trekking poles will help ensure your safety and enjoyment. If you're really testing the definition of "early season," consider packing your snowshoes, just in case. And carry all the liquid refreshment you'll need. Though you'll hear cascading water on the ascent, it's not easy to reach.

FACT

BY VEHICLE

From the Glacier Public Service Center on Hwy 542, drive east 13.1 mi (21 km). Just before the Nooksack River bridge, turn left (east) onto Road 32

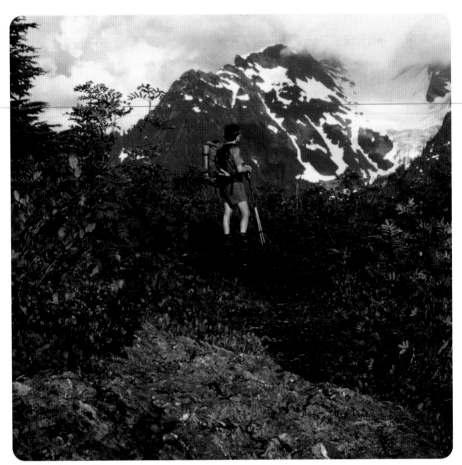

On Goat Mountain

toward Hannegan Pass. At the junction in 1.3 mi (2.1 km), stay left on Ruth Creek Road 32. Park beside the road, near the trailhead, at 2.5 mi (4 km), 2500 ft (762 m).

ON FOOT

Your destination is directly north. The frequently switchbacking trail climbs generally north-northwest, curves east higher on the mountain, then turns north again where it dwindles to a route. The ascent is extremely steep, gaining 800 ft (244 m) within the first 1 mi (0.6 km).

At 0.75 mi (1.2 km) get a peek at Mt. Shuksan (south-southeast). Enter Mount Baker Wilderness at 1.8 mi (2.9 km).

Shortly beyond the wilderness boundary sign, watch for an overgrown right **spur**. Leading southeast toward Mt. Sefrit, it ends in 0.5 mi (0.8 km) on a rocky knoll where the Goat Mtn fire lookout cabin stood until the early 1960s.

From the lookout spur, the main trail continues zigzagging upward— among heather, berry bushes, and a few mountain hemlocks.

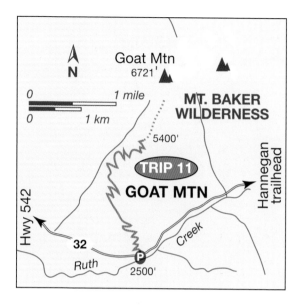

Reach **open slopes** near 2.8 mi (4.5 km), 4800 ft (1463 m). The view here is expansive and includes the summit of Mt. Baker (southwest). Because of the trail's southern exposure, hiking this far should be possible in early May.

Near 3.7 mi (6 km), after passing through vibrant pink heather, the trail briefly loses its composure. Follow whichever muddy gully appeals to you.

On a level stretch near **trail's end**—4.2 mi (6.8 km), 5450 ft (1661 m)—the vista is sufficiently compelling that most hikers drop their packs, raise their Platypus bottles, toast their good fortune, and decide this was their destination.

Church Mtn is visible west. Mt. Herman is southwest, looming over the highway. Behind it, to the right, is Mt. Baker. Mt. Shuksan is south-southeast, with Price Glacier swooping down its north slope toward Price Lake. Below (southeast) is Ruth Creek valley, with Mt. Sefrit rising above.

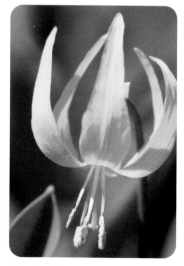

Beyond trail's end, the path dwindles to a route as it heads north, traversing grassy slopes. It all but disappears around 6000 ft (1829 m), but offers a commanding vantage well before that.

Capable scramblers, seeking further challenge and a full 360° view, don't need directions to continue to the summit ridge at 5 mi (8 km), then follow it 0.5 mi (0.8 km) northeast to the 6550-ft (1996-m) **south summit**. The nearby true summit of 6721-ft (2049-m) Goat Mtn is a technical climb.

Glacier lily

TRIP 12
HANNEGAN PEAK

LOCATION	Mt. Baker Wilderness
	Mt. Baker-Snoqualmie National Forest
ROUND TRIP	10 mi (16.1 km)
ELEVATION GAIN	3086 ft (941 m)
KEY ELEVATIONS	trailhead 3100 ft (945 m), Hannegan Pass 5100 ft (1554 m)
	Hannegan Peak 6186 ft (1885 m)
HIKING TIME	4½ to 5½ hours
DIFFICULTY	moderate
MAP	*Green Trails* Mt. Shuksan 14

OPINION

"I waited out a whole week of rain for this," our fellow summiteer said. "And you know what?" He swept his arm outward, motioning at the serrated horizon. "It was worth it." He stared a while longer in silence then quietly added, "Yup, definitely worth it."

Hannegan Peak is near Hannegan Pass, which is on the initial leg of the Copper Ridge / Whatcom Pass odyssey. But when most backpackers arrive at the pass—having hiked only the first 4 mi (6.4 km) of a 45 mi (72.4 km) circuit (Trip 42) in which they'll ascend 10,000 ft (3048 m)—they can't be bothered to drop packs and detour to the peak.

Upon recrossing the pass five days later, most backpackers again ignore the peak and scurry on, eager to tear open that bag of Cheetos they left in the car trunk, then go knock back a beer and tuck into a burger 'n fries just down the road.

They miss one of the journey's highlights, but in doing so they reserve themselves an incentive to return and dayhike to the peak. And because the trail to Hannegan Pass is easy yet scenic, re-hiking it feels like a privilege rather than a chore.

Probing Ruth Creek valley, waterfalls, avalanche greenery and snowfields are frequently in view. From the Hannegan trailhead until just shy of the pass, the grade is gentle. No need to engage your lower gears.

Hannegan Pass is clutched between buttresses of Hannegan Peak to the north and Ruth Mountain to the south. It's small, forested, and offers only a glimpse east into the headwaters of the Chilliwack River. As a destination, it's a letdown, especially after such an exceptional approach.

But Hannegan Peak is only 1120 ft (341 m) above and 1 mi (1.6 km) beyond. A well defined spur climbs from the pass to the rounded summit, where you can survey Copper Ridge and identify many of the North Cascades' most revered mountains.

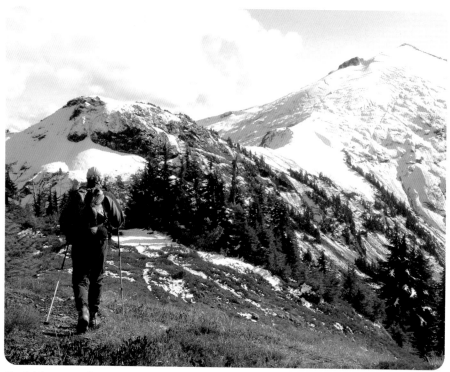

Ruth Mountain, from Hannegan Peak

In summer, Hannegan Peak also affords sanctuary from the flies that will no doubt badger you from the trailhead to the pass. Ruth Creek valley ranks high on our *Worst Infestation* list. Wear long pants and a long-sleeve shirt to help preserve your sanity while under constant attack.

FACT

BY VEHICLE

From the Glacier Public Service Center on Highway 542, drive east 13.1 mi (21.1 km). Just before the Nooksack River bridge, turn left (east) onto Road 32 toward Hannegan Pass. At the junction in 1.3 mi (2.1 km), stay left on Ruth Creek Road 32. At 5.4 mi (8.7 km) reach the road's end campground and trailhead, at 3100 ft (945 m). On weekends, expect to see dozens of vehicles here. The tentsites are between the parking lot and Ruth Creek.

ON FOOT

The trail is initially level. It leads east, gradually curving southeast, following Ruth Creek upstream.

Within ten minutes, the steep cliffs of Mt. Sefrit and Nooksack Ridge are visible right (south) across the valley. Continue through beautiful, mature, mountain-hemlock forest with occasional views.

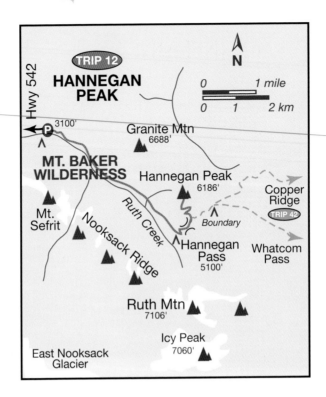

At 3 mi (5 km), 4000 ft (1220 m) the ascent begins in earnest. About 1½ hours from the trailhead, a right spur drops to a creeklet then rises to **Hannegan camp** on a knoll. Visible south is glacier dolloped, 7106-ft (2166-m) Ruth Mtn. The main trail begins a switchbacking ascent generally north, but refill water bottles before continuing. The pass and the peak are dry.

Fifteen minutes above the campground, enter 5100-ft (1554-m) **Hannegan Pass** at 4 mi (6.4 km) and reach a junction. The main trail proceeds straight, contouring briefly before switchbacking generally east, down into the headwater drainage of the Chilliwack River. Right is a climbers' route curving south toward Ruth Mtn. Turn left (northwest) for Hannegan Peak.

Heading generally north, ascend 1120 ft (341 m) in 1 mi (1.6 km) through open forest, steep meadow, more trees, then heather. Reach the comfortably broad summit of 6186-ft (1885-m) **Hannegan Peak** at 5 mi (8 km). Fit hikers top out about 2½ hours after departing the trailhead.

The panorama includes Goat Mtn northwest, Mt. Larrabee north-northwest, Slesse Mtn north in Canada, Mt. Redoubt east-northeast, Mt. Challenger southeast, Ruth Mtn south, Mt. Shuksan south-southwest, and Mt. Baker southwest.

TRIP 13
TABLE MOUNTAIN

LOCATION	Heather Meadows Recreation Area Mt. Baker Wilderness
ROUND TRIP	1 to 3 mi (1.6 to 5 km)
ELEVATION GAIN	600 ft (183 m)
KEY ELEVATIONS	trailhead 5100 ft (1554 m), Table Mtn 5700 ft (1737 m)
HIKING TIME	1 to 2 hours
DIFFICULTY	easy
MAP	*Green Trails* Mt. Shuksan 14

OPINION

Most people who drive up Mt. Baker to Artist Point don't hike. They think the parking lot is the destination. But looming directly above is a rocky mesa offering the shortest premier trail in the North Cascades.

Table Mtn's 360° panorama is a head spinner. The glimmer twins—Mounts Baker and Shuksan—are seemingly within spitting distance. The Border Peaks are also nearby, straddling the imaginary line between the U.S. and Canada.

Because the summit is as flat as its namesake, you can wander. Huge rock slabs beckon in all directions. The eye-popping overlooks are as compelling as the peak-studded horizon. Pick your way out to the edge of the escarpment and peer over.

Traversing the mountaintop initially looks easy, but the way becomes indefinite and requires light scrambling. Permanent snowfields mean the trail is never evident for its entire length. Where it's obscured by snow, follow cairns or perhaps the bootprints of previous hikers. If you find no joy in navigating rough terrain, turn around when the route gets sketchy.

Avoid crowds by hopping onto the Table before 10 a.m. or after 6 p.m. Mt. Shuksan is most photogenic at dusk.

FACT

BY VEHICLE

From the Glacier Public Service Center on Hwy 542, drive east 25 mi (40.2 km) to the Artist Point parking lot on Kulshan Ridge. The highway—entirely paved—ends here, at 5100 ft (1554 m). The snowpack will probably prevent you from driving that far until late July. In anticipation of winter storms, the road crew closes the highway again in mid-September.

ON FOOT

The trail departs the southwest side of the parking lot (nearest Mt. Baker). There's an immediate choice, not shown on maps. Take the trail on the right, behind the large trailhead sign. It immediately ascends the lava cliffs of Table Mtn.

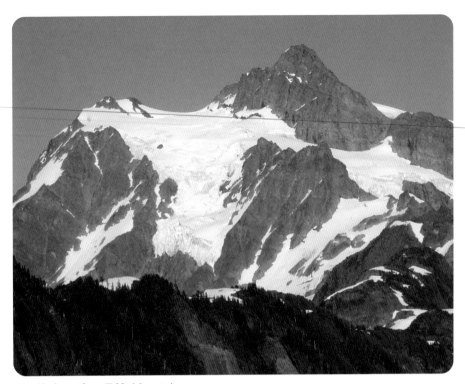

Mt. Shuksan, from Table Mountain

Reach the top at 0.4 mi (0.6 km), 5700 ft (1737 m). Before proceeding, digress to the southeast periphery for the optimal view of Mt. Shuksan (east-southeast). Then follow the main trail west along the plateau's south rim. Mt. Baker looms southwest.

Diverging paths beckon. The main trail ends at about 1.5 mi (2.4 km). Beyond, let curiosity and instinct be your guide, but stay oriented while you wonder and be cautious on the icy snow and near the mountain's precipitous edges.

To the northwest you can overlook Iceberg and Hayes lakes. To the northeast you can peer into the valley cupping Bagley Lakes.

Return the way you came: via the trail on Table Mtn's east end.

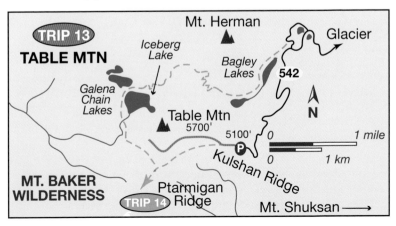

PTARMIGAN RIDGE

LOCATION	Mt. Baker Wilderness
ROUND TRIP	9.4 mi (15.1 km) to Coleman Pinnacle
ELEVATION GAIN	1000 ft (305 m)
KEY ELEVATIONS	trailhead 5100 ft (1554 m)
	near Coleman Pinnacle 6100 ft (1859 m)
HIKING TIME	3½ to 6 hours
DIFFICULTY	moderate
MAP	*Green Trails* Mt. Shuksan 14

OPINION

Winter weather at high altitude can be so sharply cold it's painful, even frightening, like the clutch of a mugger. And in the North Cascades, the snow accompanying that cold often falls with apocalyptic intensity—hence the ponderous glaciers that still drape the region's dominant peaks.

So those few, late-summer days when sustained alpine-zone hiking is not only possible but enjoyable—blue sky, hot sun, gravel rather than ice crunching beneath your boots—are immeasurably precious.

To wrest every ounce of joy from such a day, rouse yourself early, drive Hwy 542 to Artist Point and hike Ptarmigan Ridge, where the views are vast, the beauty is raw, and the stupendous scenery bears no resemblance to the tame, humdrum settings where most of us spend our days.

Snow-free tread permitting, hike at least 3.5 mi (5.6 km) before turning back. In addition to the postcard image of Mt. Baker and the Rainbow Glacier, you'll see Mt. Blum, Mt. Hagan, Mt. Bacon, Mt. Shuksan, and numerous other titans. En route, you'll cross meltwater creeklets singing their soothing watersongs. You'll pass pockets of flourishing wildflowers. And you'll be eyed with bemusement by the resident marmots and pikas.

Beyond Coleman Pinnacle, the trail skims across talus slopes and snowpatches, winds through a bouldery moonscape, and deposits you at the Sholes Glacier, all the while offering ever more staggering vistas and an increasingly intimate encounter with Mt. Baker. Continue as far as the weather, the snowpack, your experience, and common sense will allow. The farther you go, the better it gets.

Just don't cross steep snowfields without an ice axe and the know-how to self-arrest. Don't risk getting stuck on a distant ridge when cloud or fog might diminish visibility. And don't wander blithely onto the glacier, where hidden crevasses await the unwary.

Upon arrival at Artist Point, expect to be as disheartened by the crowd as you are elated by the mountainous panorama. Bear in mind, most people don't stray far from their vehicles, and many who set foot on the trail turn back within a mile. Stride on. You'll soon shake the sightseers.

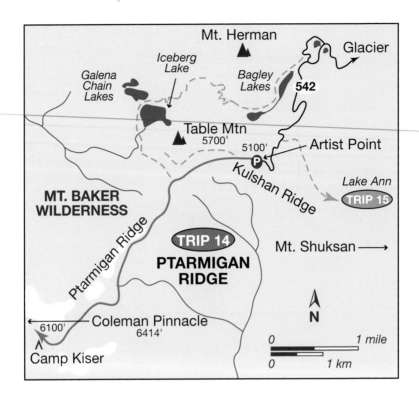

FACT

BY VEHICLE

From the Glacier Public Service Center on Hwy 542, drive east 25 mi (40.2 km) to the Artist Point parking lot on Kulshan Ridge. The highway— entirely paved—ends here, at 5100 ft (1554 m). The snowpack will probably prevent you from driving that far until late July. In anticipation of winter storms, the road crew closes the highway again in mid-September.

ON FOOT

The trail departs the southwest side of the parking lot (nearest Mt. Baker). There's an immediate choice, not shown on maps.

Don't take the trail on the right ascending the lava cliffs of Table Mtn. Instead, follow Galena Chain Lakes trail 682 west-northwest.

Ignore a rough, right spur ascending Table Mtn at 0.2 mi (0.3 km). Your trail remains mostly level, contouring southwest. At 1.2 mi (1.9 km), 5200 ft (1585 m), the Galena Chain Lakes loop forks right (northwest). Go left (south) for Ptarmigan Ridge.

Descend into a basin, where the trail splits temporarily. Either fork will do; they soon rejoin to form a better-defined trail on the beginning of **Ptarmigan Ridge**, up to your left.

Follow the ridge trail upward, then left across a steep, airy, south-facing slope of rock, scree, volcanic dust, and possibly snow. The vistas expand the farther you walk.

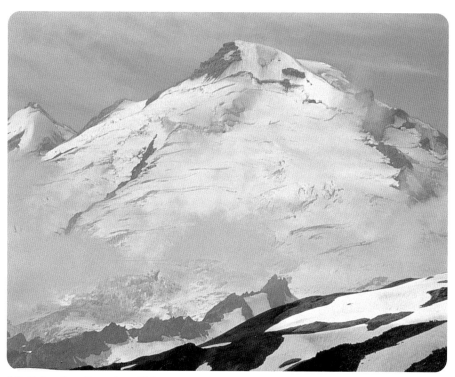

Mt. Baker, from Ptarmigan Ridge

At 3.7 mi (6 km), 5600 ft (1707 km), Mt. Baker's Rainbow Glacier is visible. The trail then heads southwest 1 mi (1.6 km), ascending 500 ft (152 m) to the slopes of **Coleman Pinnacle**.

Backpacking? You'll find flat, bare tentsites beneath the pinnacle, but you'll be relying on snowmelt unless you hauled sufficient water.

How far you can safely hike the Ptarmigan Ridge trail—especially beyond Coleman Pinnacle—depends on the snowpack, your level of experience and preparation, and the weather.

During late summer or early autumn, in years of low snowfall, a trail will be evident continuing west past Coleman Pinnacle, to the **Sholes Glacier**.

Just before the trail turns sharply northwest beneath Coleman Pinnacle, a southward cross-country descent is also possible: to an icy, turquoise tarn 0.6 mi (1 km) distant and about 400 ft (122 m) below.

TRIP 15
LAKE ANN

LOCATION	Mt. Baker Wilderness
ROUND TRIP	8.2 mi (13.2 km) to saddle above lake
ELEVATION GAIN	1700 ft (518 m)
KEY ELEVATIONS	trailhead 4700 ft (1433 m), lowpoint 3900 ft (1189 m) saddle above lake 4800 ft (1463 m)
HIKING TIME	3 to 4 hours
DIFFICULTY	easy
MAP	*Green Trails* Mt. Shuksan 14

OPINION

The perfect hiking boots are hard to find, because they're a fusion of conflicting attributes: light but stiff. The perfect hike is equally rare because it too is a contradiction: easy but scenic. The Lake Ann trail, however, comes close to achieving that tricky balance. Without taxing your stamina, it lofts you as close as a mere hiker can get to the immense, daunting Mt. Shuksan.

Driving to such a high-elevation trailhead, then immediately descending on the trail, is odd. Plunge in anyway. The initial drop through lush forest leads to an idyllic hanging valley—the headwaters of Swift Creek. En route, you might hear the thunderous roar of an ice chunk breaking off a glacier and crasching down a rock face.

After skimming through grass and flowers, the trail dodges a few more trees then begins climbing to the saddle above Lake Ann. The highlights: heather meadows, creeklets cascading in all directions, and tiny, graceful ferns softening the otherwise stark boulder field beneath the saddle.

The final ascent to the saddle is steep, but there's no shortage of boulders inviting you to stop, sit, rest, and meditate upon the surrounding beauty, or— if you're shod in the latest flashy-but-flimsy offering from the fashion-obsessed outdoor footwear industry—massage your feet.

Fast hikers can reach Lake Ann in 1½ hours, but that's not where this short journey climaxes. Instead of descending from the saddle to the lake, find the climbers' path veering up to the left and go marvel at Lower Curtis Glacier on Mt. Shuksan.

FACT

BY VEHICLE

From the Glacier Public Service Center on Hwy 542, drive east 23 mi (37 km)—entirely on pavement. The trailhead and parking area are on the left, at 4700 ft (1433 km), midway between Austin Pass picnic area and road's end at Artist Point. The snowpack will probably prevent you from driving that far

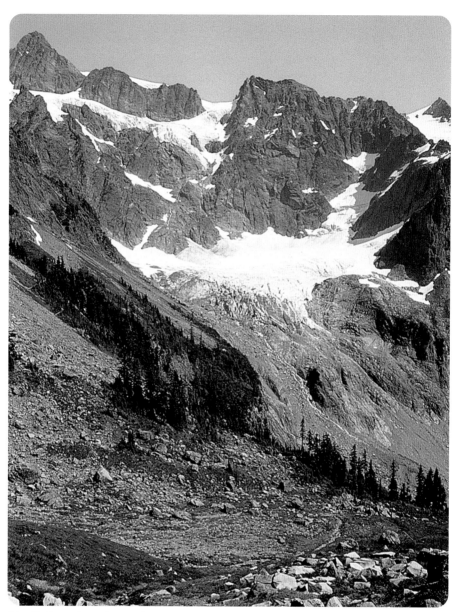

Mt. Shuksan, from above Lake Ann

until late July. In anticipation of winter storms, the road crew closes the highway again in mid-September.

ON FOOT

From the alpine trailhead, begin an 800-ft (244-m) descent, initially east then southeast. Re-enter forest at 1.4 mi (2.2 km).

At 2.3 mi (3.7 km), 3900 ft (1189 m), the trail pops out of the forest, into stream-fed **meadows**. Arrive at a junction. Bear left for Lake Ann. The right fork careens into the depths of Swift Creek canyon.

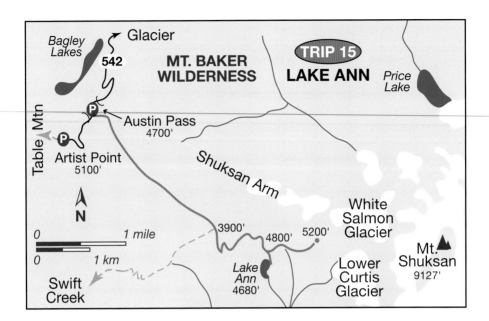

From the junction, ascend south-southeast, then northeast, to the **saddle** at 4.1 mi (6.6 km), 4800 ft (1463 m). **Lake Ann**—frozen most of the year—is visible 120 ft (37 m) below (south).

Either continue down the trail to the shore, or fork left onto a rough, narrow **climbers' path** leading generally east 0.7 mi (1.1 km) toward Fisher Chimney—a popular route for climbers attempting to summit Mt. Shuksan. The path gets precarious before ending at 5200 ft (1585 m).

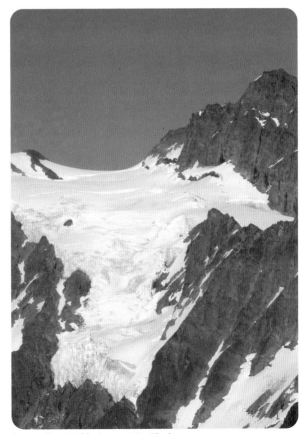

Lower Curtis Glacier on Mt. Shuksan

RAINBOW RIDGE

LOCATION	Mt. Baker Wilderness
ROUND TRIP	4.4 mi (7.1 km)
ELEVATION GAIN	1200 ft (366 m)
KEY ELEVATIONS	trailhead 3600 ft (1097 m), highpoint 4800 ft (1463 m)
HIKING TIME	2½ to 3½ hours
DIFFICULTY	easy
MAPS	*Green Trails* Mt. Shuksan 14
	Mt. Baker 13 (to identify glaciers)
	Lake Shannon 46 (shows lower reaches of Road 1130)

OPINION

Ice-armored leviathans everywhere you look, including the preeminent Mounts Baker and Shuksan. A 2000-ft (610-m) cascade plunging into Rainbow Creek. The glaciated chaos of Avalanche Gorge. And in the center of it all, a trail surges through parklands to a lonesome ridge, vast vistas, and infinite inspiration.

The Rainbow Ridge trail has been ignored by cartographers, but looking at a map you can fathom the course it follows from road's end: generally northwest, between Marten Lake (southwest) and Rainbow Creek (northeast).

The trail's relative obscurity ensures you won't encounter a throng of hikers here, like at Ptarmigan Ridge or Park Butte. The first 50 yd/m are sketchy and rough. After that, the trail is decent all the way up the ridge and a short way along the crest. It'll make you sweat, but only briefly.

Though short, Rainbow Ridge warrants backpacking. Potential campsites are numerous and scenic. A smart plan is to begin hiking about 6 p.m., when the cool of the evening calms the flies and makes exertion more pleasant. In late summer, you'll still have plenty of daylight to pitch your tent. Then you can sit outside and enjoy the view without flapping furiously at the flies. After witnessing Shuksan at sunset and Baker at sunrise, wander the ridge out and back, then leave by 10 a.m., before the flies rev up.

FACT

BY VEHICLE

Drive Hwy 20 east 16.5 mi (26.6 km) from Sedro Woolley, or west 6 mi (9.7 km) from Concrete. Turn north onto the Grandy-Baker Lake Road. At 17.8 mi (28.7 km) you'll see Boulder Creek campground on the right. Pass it, cross the creek, and 0.2 mi (0.3 km) farther turn left (north) onto Marten Lake Road 1130. Reset your trip odometer to zero.

At 1.5 mi (2.4 km) fork right. Cross a creek at 2.1 mi (3.4 km). At the signed junction in 3.9 mi (6.3 km), go left (northwest) toward Rainbow Falls. At 4.5 mi

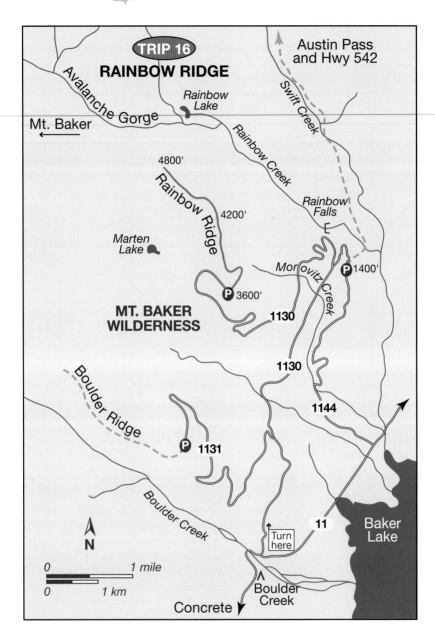

TRIP 16
RAINBOW RIDGE

(7.2 km), check out Rainbow Falls on the right. Reach a fork 9.5 mi (15.3 km) from the Baker Lake Road. The road ends here in a clearcut, at 3600 ft (1097 m). Park in the flat area to the right. The rougher road left leads to the trail.

ON FOOT

The rough road ends abruptly. Continue in the same direction, picking your way over deadfall and through shoulder-high brush. Then angle right, entering forest spared from the saw. The route might still be flagged. A **trail** becomes apparent within 0.2 mi (0.3 km) of the rough road.

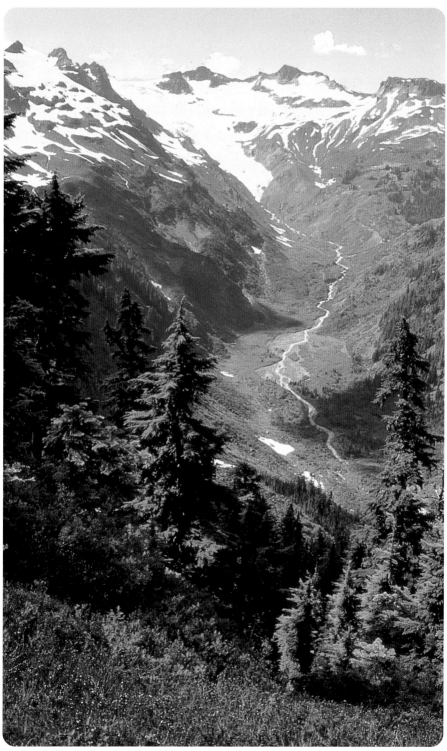

Avalanche Gorge, from Rainbow Ridge

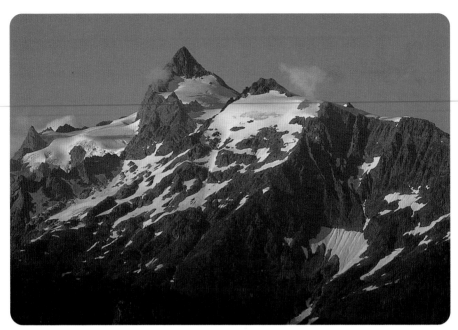

Mt. Shuksan, from the road to Rainbow Ridge trailhead

Emerge from timber into heather and stunted trees. Heading north-northwest, reach a small **meadow**, then resume the steep ascent. Gain the ridgecrest at 1.2 mi (1.9 km), 4200 ft (1280 m).

Atop the ridge, follow the trail northwest, through heather and blueberry bushes, among large boulders, past tall mountain hemlocks. At about 2.2 mi (3.5 km), 4800 ft (1280 m) you can peer into **Avalanche Gorge** 2000 ft (610 m) below (north).

You've hiked Ptarmigan Ridge? If so, you'll enjoy identifying it from here. It's visible northwest, slicing under the base of a green knob and reddish slope, right of a mesa.

Beyond 2.2 mi (3.5 km), the trail descends the south side of Rainbow Ridge. Follow the undulating tread as far as you feel comfortable doing so; it eventually diminishes to a game path. Potential tentsites abound.

Mt. Baker's Rainbow Glacier is visible west. Mt. Shuksan's Sulphide Glacier is northeast. To the southeast, Hagan Mtn, Anderson Butte and Mt. Watson are in front of Bacon Glacier on Bacon Peak.

RAILROAD GRADE / PARK BUTTE

LOCATION	Mt. Baker National Recreation Area
ROUND TRIP	8 mi (12.9 km) to High camp on RR Grade
	6.6 mi (10.6 km) to Park Butte
ELEVATION GAIN	2900 ft (884 m) to High camp on RR Grade
	2100 ft (640 m) to Park Butte
KEY ELEVATIONS	trailhead 3300 ft (1006 m)
	High camp on RR Grade 6200 ft (1890 m)
	Park Butte 5400 ft (1646 m)
HIKING TIME	4 to 5 hours for High camp on RR Grade, 3 hours for
	Park Butte, 5 to 7 hours for both
DIFFICULTY	moderate for either, challenging for both
MAPS	*Green Trails* Hamilton 45, Lake Shannon 46 (shows Road 12)

OPINION

Railroad Grade and Park Butte are veritable holy sites—slightly less crowded than those of most religions but no less moving if your place of worship is the mountains.

Your time is limited? Chug up Railroad (RR) Grade. Given a full day, robust hikers can pay homage to both RR Grade and Park Butte. You have two days? Devote the first to RR Grade, the second to Park Butte and the Scott Paul trail.

Most hikers manage to go at least part way up RR Grade—a long, gentle moraine. The raw beauty of Mt. Baker towering above lush meadows motivates many to exceed their usual limitations. See photo on page 4. Suddenly you'll peek over the moraine at the roaring chaos of Rocky Creek in the gorge beneath Easton Glacier. It's as if you're witnessing another, much younger planet.

On weekends, RR Grade feels like a pilgrimage route for pantheists. But an atmosphere of awe and reverence tends to prevail, making a conga line a bit more tolerable. Just don't be lured onto the ice, even if you see others there, unless you have the skill and equipment to negotiate those yawning chasms.

After the RR Grade trail peters out, you can continue wending your way upward through rock and rubble. Footprints in the sand between rocks offer hints of a route. Scramblers can navigate the tantalizing reaches beside Easton Glacier all the way to High camp near 6200 ft (1890 m), beyond which crampons and an ice axe are necessary. Gazing up at Mt. Baker from High camp, the summit seems within easy reach, but it takes climbers another five hours.

At High camp's rocky perch next to the cascading ice, you can pitch your tent with glacier travelers. Hauling a full pack up there is a grind, but the rewards include an astounding view of ice and ocean. You'll see not only Easton Glacier, but the San Juan Islands.

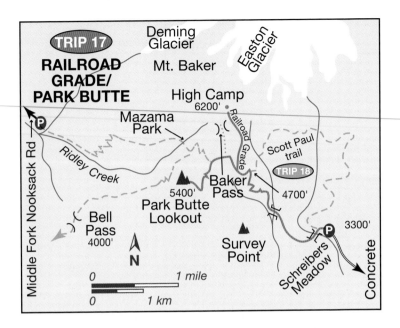

If you make it to High camp, cross the small snowfield west to another rocky outcrop and get a staggering view of the Deming Glacier. It's difficult to believe any view could compete with what you've seen already, but this one does. Approach cautiously. The rock is straining to answer the call of gravity.

Hiking to Park Butte feels less adventurous than ascending RR Grade, but it too offers a visual feast. Mt. Baker appears even larger here, and you'll overlook your ascent route. Also visible are Deming Glacier, the canyon below the Black Buttes, and the impressive Sisters Range.

Atop the butte is a former fire lookout cabin maintained by the Skagit Alpine Club of Mt. Vernon (www.skagitalpineclub.com) and open to the public. Treat it as if you're a guest, which you in fact are.

In and above Morovitz Meadow, paths radiate to points other than the area's two popular destinations. Dayhikers should ignore them. RR Grade and Park Butte are more rewarding.

FACT

BY VEHICLE

Drive Hwy 20 east 16.5 mi (26.6 km) from Sedro Woolley, or west 6 mi (10 km) from Concrete. Turn north onto Grandy-Baker Lake Road and reset your trip odometer to zero. Proceed northeast 12.4 mi (20 km). Just past Rocky Creek bridge, go left (northwest) on South Fork Nooksack Road 12. Ignore the unsigned right fork at 14.2 mi (22.9 km). At 15.9 mi (25.6 km) turn right onto Sulphur Creek Road 13, signed for Mt. Baker National Rec Area. Follow signs to Shriebers Meadow. Reach the trailhead parking lot at 21.1 mi (34 km), 3300 ft (1006 m).

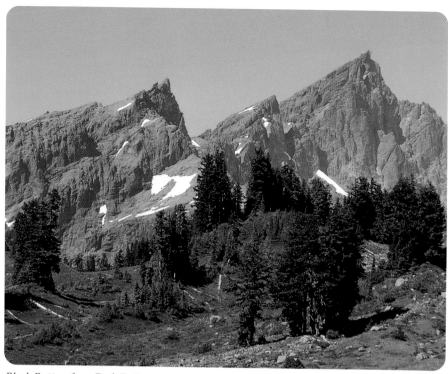

Black Buttes, from Park Butte

ON FOOT

The trail departs right of the info kiosk. Within a couple minutes, ignore the signed Scott Paul trail forking right. Cross the bridge spanning **Sulphur Creek**.

Proceed on stretches of boardwalk through pond-splattered Shriebers Meadow: southwest, gradually curving northwest into forest.

At 1 mi (1.6 km) cross a rubble-strewn expanse where meltwater torrents from Easton Glacier occasionally rearrange the scenery. Cross a suspension bridge over **Rocky Creek**, re-enter forest, and begin a switchbacking ascent northwest.

Just before reaching **lower Morovitz Meadow**, the Scott Paul trail forks right at 1.9 mi (3.1 km), 4700 ft (1433 m). It loops over moraine and meadow back to the trailhead. Bear left for RR Grade.

Reach a junction at 2 mi (3.2 km), 4800 ft (1463 m), in lower Morovitz Meadow. Left leads to Park Butte, whose crowning lookout cabin is visible above (west-southwest). Right leads north to RR Grade.

Heading for RR Grade, ascend a long flight of stone steps. Soon pass about eight treed tentsites, some with views of the looming volcano. Beyond the tentsites, begin ascending the crest of the **RR Grade moraine**.

Near 5400 ft (1646 m), 3 mi (5 km), the RR Grade trail dwindles to a climbers' path. It's another 1 mi (1.6 km) generally north over jumbled rock to **High camp** at 6200 ft (1890 m), near the edge of Easton Glacier.

Turning left at the 2-mi (3-km) junction in lower Morovitz Meadow, hike northwest to another junction at 2.3 mi (3.7 km). Here, in the **upper meadow**,

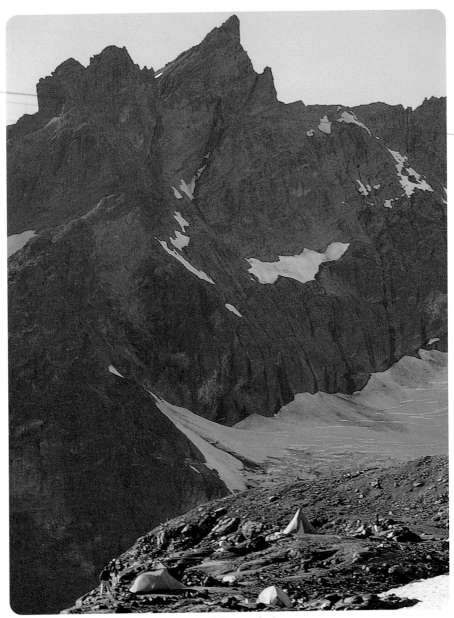

Hiker-accessible camp between Deming and Easton glaciers

the left fork ascends southwest 1 mi (1.6 km) to the summit of 5400-ft (1646-km) **Park Butte**. The optimal Mt. Baker vantage is from the tarn on the side of Park Butte. Look for a spur 200 ft (60 m) below the lookout cabin.

Right at the 2.3-mi (3.7-km) junction in the upper meadow descends generally northwest to Mazama Park at 3 mi (4.8 km), 4400 ft (1341 m). If the subalpine campsites just north of the RR Grade junction are full, you'll likely find a vacancy and perhaps total privacy in Mazama Park.

TRIP 18
SCOTT PAUL

LOCATION	Mt. Baker Wilderness
LOOP	7.9 mi (12.7 km)
ELEVATION GAIN	1800 ft (550 m)
KEY ELEVATIONS	trailhead 3300 ft (1006 m), highpoint 5000 ft (1524 m)
HIKING TIME	3½ to 5 hours
DIFFICULTY	moderate
MAPS	*Green Trails* Hamilton 45, Lake Shannon 46 (shows Road 12)

Here's yet another way to scurry onto the flanks of mighty Mt. Baker. A relatively new trail, finished in 1994, it was named after the ranger who kept the project alive until his death in 1993.

Although not as wondrous as nearby Railroad Grade, the Scott Paul trail is exceptionally scenic and enjoyable. If you have two days for this area, hike Railroad Grade one day, then combine Scott Paul and Park Butte the next.

The Scott Paul trail is wide, well-graded and smooth, with extensive ditches to control erosion—a veritable Yellow Brick Road. Initially it climbs through a pleasant forest punctuated by grand trees—some of them 5 yd/m in circumference. Moss garlands and baby's breath lighten the atmosphere. Then you suddenly reach an open saddle and a new perspective of Mounts Baker and Shuksan.

Tall grass, luscious berry patches in season, and a calming view of sweeping virgin forests below make the saddle an excellent rest stop or picnic destination, especially if you have small children or aren't feeling ambitious. Moderate-paced walkers arrive at the saddle in just over an hour. Unfortunately, on hot days between mid-July and late August, flies can be a deterrent to extended relaxation.

Continuing, the trail climbs briefly then relents, providing a couple miles of level hiking. It weaves in and out of meadowy gullies, crossing several creeklets and staying mostly in the open. Flower gardens and tiny ferns flourish in the fertile volcanic soil.

Eventually, you plunge into the gorge below Easton Glacier. This rocky, dusty, desolate stretch resembles northern Arizona. Even the smell is reminiscent of sand and salt cedars in Southwest riparian regions. And the vast gorge itself—roaring river below, ice and rubble above—could be in Ladakh. The suspension bridge (thankfully, far more stable than those on third-world trekking routes) contributes to the exotic atmosphere.

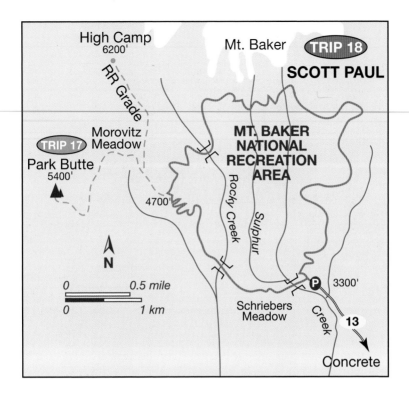

FACT

BY VEHICLE

Drive Hwy 20 east 16.5 mi (26.6 km) from Sedro Woolley, or west 6 mi (9.7 km) from Concrete. Turn north onto Grandy-Baker Lake Road and reset your trip odometer to zero. Proceed northeast 12.4 mi (20 km). Just past Rocky Creek bridge, go left (northwest) on South Fork Nooksack Road 12. Ignore the unsigned right fork at 14.2 mi (22.9 km). At 15.9 mi (25.6 km) turn right onto Sulphur Creek Road 13, signed for Mt. Baker National Rec Area. Follow signs to Shriebers Meadow. Reach the trailhead parking lot at 21.1 mi (34 km), 3300 ft (1006 m).

ON FOOT

The trail departs right of the info kiosk. Within a couple minutes, fork right onto the signed Scott Paul trail. Straight, across the bridge spanning Sulphur Creek, leads to Railroad Grade and Park Butte.

Ascend 1400 ft (427 m) in 2 mi (3.2 km) through forest to an open, grassy 4700-ft (1433-m) **saddle**, with views of Mt. Baker (left / north), and Mt. Shuksan (right / northeast). From the saddle, ascend moderately northeast, then north to about 5000 ft (1524 m). The trail then contours northwest.

Soon cross **Sulphur Creek**. Near 5.25 mi (8.4 km), go southwest and cross **Metcalf Moraine**. The trail then drops into the gorge below Easton Glacier.

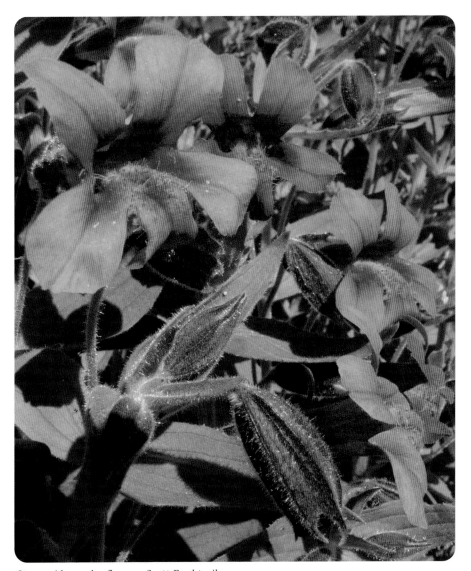

Streamside monkeyflowers, Scott Paul trail

Cross the suspension bridge over **Rocky Creek** at 5.5 mi (8.9 km), then ascend the south end of the moraine. The Railroad Grade trail is above, on the moraine crest.

Reach a junction at 6 mi (9.7 km). Left descends 1.9 mi (3.1 km) generally southeast to the trailhead. Right (northwest) leads to Railroad Grade and Park Butte.

Time and energy permitting, scoot up to Park Butte Lookout before looping back to the trailhead. This 2.8-mi (4.5-km) round-trip detour will increase your total distance to 10.7 mi (17.2 km) and your total elevation gain to 3200 ft (975 m).

TRIP 19

THORNTON LAKES / TRAPPERS PEAK

LOCATION	Ross Lake NRA / North Cascades National Park
ROUND TRIP	10.6 mi (17.1 km) to Trappers Peak
ELEVATION GAIN	3364 ft (1025 m) to peak
KEY ELEVATIONS	trailhead 2600 ft (792 m), overlook 4960 ft (1512 m)
	peak 5964 ft (1818 m)
HIKING TIME	4½ to 5½ hours
DIFFICULTY	moderate
MAP	*Green Trails* Marblemount 47

Greed is maligned. It's not always bad. In the mountains, greed can be admirable. Desire to see more, hike farther, climb higher, wring a little more adventure from the day—these are virtues. So don't be satisfied at Thornton Lakes. Be greedy. Go farther, to Trappers Peak.

The overlook above Thornton Lakes is rewarding, but the trail probes unimpressive forest all the way there. Beyond, the route is a fun challenge above treeline. Atop Trappers, the panorama is complete, and you'll exult in the accomplishment.

Backpacking here allows experienced scramblers time to explore the middle and upper lakes and the tantalizing, rocky terrain northwest of the lower lake. But don't expect a cush campsite; the sites at the lower lake, just across the outlet stream, are not pleasant.

If dayhiking, don't drop to the lakes. Find a perch on the huge boulders, high above the lower lake. From here, you can see the lower two lakes in the cirque beneath looming Mt. Triumph. You can also set your sights on Trappers Peak—northeast above the first lake. It's not as difficult to summit as it appears. In the other direction, past the highway, Teebone Ridge and the Newhalem Creek drainage are visible. The Neve Glacier, Pyramid Peak, and Colonial Peak are east.

After you've savored that spectacle, continue up Trappers Peak. Don't let 1000 ft (305 m) separate you from this trip's scenic and geographic zenith. The astounding view encompasses the wild Picket Range, the secretive, uppermost Thornton Lake, and the village of Newhalem far below (southeast).

Though the road to this trailhead is steep and rough, low-clearance cars can make it with a little coaxing. Low-energy cars must maintain speed. Think of having to gain all that elevation on foot—that'll bolster your determination behind the wheel.

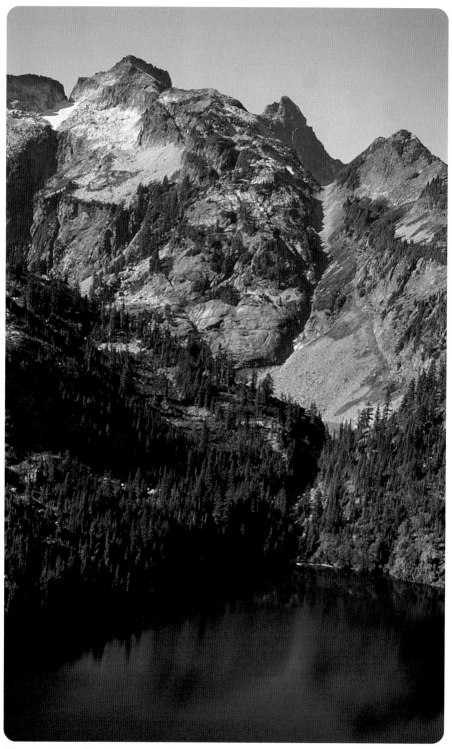

Thornton Lakes, from Trappers Peak

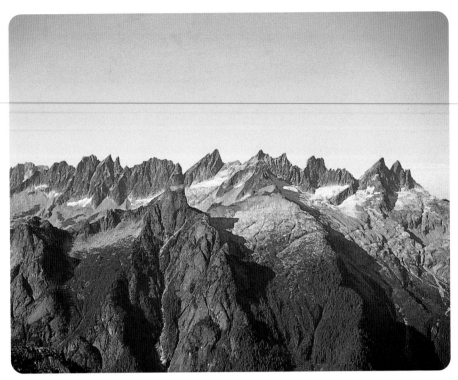

The Pickets, from Trappers Peak

FACT

BY VEHICLE

Drive Hwy 20 northeast 11 mi (17.7 km) from Marblemount, or southwest 3 mi (4.8 km) from Newhalem. Between mileposts 117 and 118, turn northwest onto the signed, unpaved Thornton Creek Road. Follow it 5.1 mi (8.2 km) to the trailhead, at 2600 ft (792 m).

ON FOOT

The trail initially heads northwest. The first 2.3 mi (3.7 km) are on a 1960s logging road—now so narrow and overgrown it looks like a trail. A mix of Douglas fir, Pacific silver fir, hemlock, cedar, alder, and maples are slowly returning.

After contouring into, then east-southeast out of the Thornton Creek drainage, the trail turns north and climbs steadily. Pass the signed national-park boundary and surmount treeline.

Reach a signed fork at 4.7 mi (7.6 km), 4960 ft (1512 m). Left leads five minutes through boulders to the **Thornton Lakes overlook**. It then continues west, descending 460 ft (140 m) in 0.6 mi (1 km) to lower Thornton Lake at 4500 ft (1372 m), where you'll find three tentsites near the outlet stream. From there, a primitive path leads north to the upper lakes.

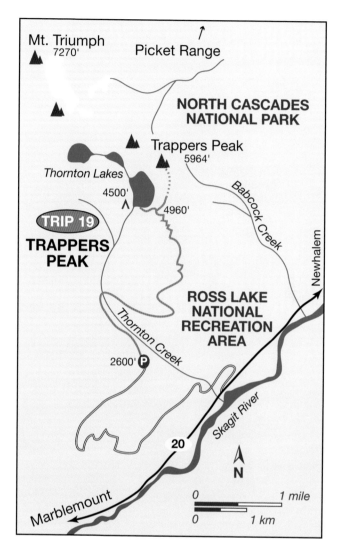

Aiming for the peak? Return to the signed fork. Proceed toward the triangular rock. A very steep but clearly defined route follows the ridgecrest generally north. The first ten minutes are the hardest. You might need to use your hands, but you'll face no exposure.

About 45 minutes after departing the signed fork, crest the 5964-ft (1818-m) summit of **Trappers Peak** at 5.3 mi (8.5 km). The shark's mouth peaks to the north comprise the Picket Range.

TRIP 20
SOURDOUGH MOUNTAIN

LOCATION	Ross Lake NRA / North Cascades National Park
ROUND TRIP	11 mi (17.7 km)
ELEVATION GAIN	5085 ft (1550 m)
KEY ELEVATIONS	trailhead 900 ft (274 m), summit 5985 ft (1824 m)
HIKING TIME	5 to 7½ hours
DIFFICULTY	challenging
MAP	*Green Trails* Diablo Dam 48

OPINION

Life: if you do it right, it's exhausting. Remember that truth when you arrive in Diablo, you gaze 5085 ft (1550 m) up at Sourdough Mtn, and your knees buckle. Because the summit affords a panorama and sense of achievement that more than compensate for the merciless ascent.

On our most recent trip, we met hikers turning back, spent and disappointed. Only three others summitted that day: a pair of marathoners training between races, and a professional photographer/climber seeking the ultimate viewpoint for his tripod.

The short switchbacks climb relentlessly through forest as ugly as it gets in the North Cascades. The spindly trees are just enough to obscure views most of the way up, yet insufficient to provide shade. It can get sizzling hot here on a sunny day, so start hiking early. Heat, however, is only a possibility. Boredom is a certainty. Unless you bring entertaining companions, you'll find little to alleviate the monotony of toiling up the mountain.

So Sourdough is the most grueling hike in this book. But the culminating vista is arguably the most spectacular a mere hiker can attain in the North Cascades. It's downright soul awakening, which is why you must go. Just keep telling yourself: the view will be worth it. Because the scenery *is* dazzling, and it's enhanced by the wave of relief and pride that'll wash over you upon striding up to the fire lookout on top.

On a clear day (otherwise forget it!) all of North Cascades National Park will be spread out before you. Big, bold, bare Jack Mtn towers above the east shore of Ross Lake. Mt. Buckner and the Boston Glacier are way south. Mt. Terror and McMillan Spire loom northwest, with Azure Lake clutched in an icy, rocky cirque below. Mt. Prophet is north. But there are hundreds more peaks visible in all directions. Anyone stationed in the Sourdough Mtn fire lookout must have felt they'd been sent to heaven—or feared they would be when lightning jolted their sky-scraping perch.

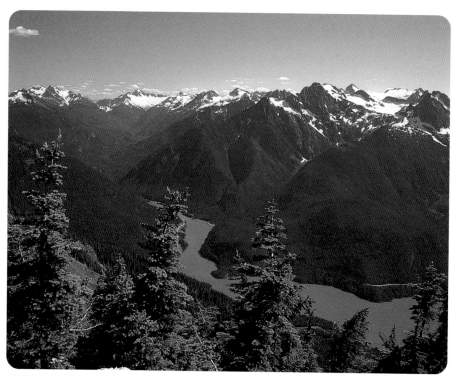

Diablo Lake far below Sourdough Mountain

Asking at the Newhalem or Marblemount park offices about trail conditions, you might be excited to hear the Sourdough trail is clear of snow to 5000 ft (1524 m) in early June. Don't go yet. That's not high enough. You need to hike 1000 ft (305 m) higher to attain the scenic reward that makes the trip worthwhile. True, Sourdough is snow-free before most high-elevation options, but assaulting it early in the season is unwise. Build up to it.

Having paid extravagantly to get there, leaving the summit is painful—emotionally at first, then physically. It's probably more punishing than the ascent. Carry trekking poles to alleviate knee strain.

FACT

BY VEHICLE

Drive Hwy 20 to the Diablo-townsite turnoff. It's 5.1 mi (8.2 km) northeast of Newhalem's east edge, or 4.3 mi (6.9 km) northwest of Colonial Creek campground on Diablo Lake. From the west side of the highway bridge spanning Gorge Lake, proceed northeast into Diablo townsite. Continue past the homes, to the domed public swimming pool. Park on the gravel shoulder paralleling the river, at 900 ft (274 m). Look across the lawn. Near the hillside you'll see the signed trailhead.

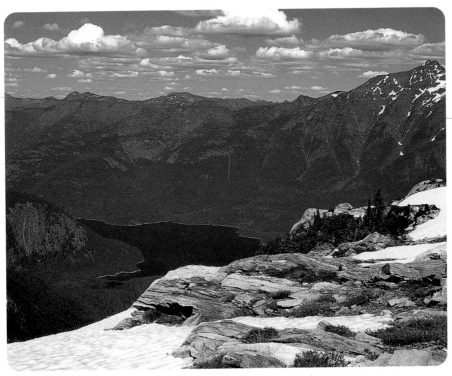

Jack Mountain rising above Ross Lake, from Sourdough Mountain

ON FOOT

Your general direction of travel is initially north. The trail switchbacks persistently for 3 mi (5 km). The first mile is on the west side of a buttress—shaded until noontime. Then the trail turns northeast into the heat of the sun. The forest is dry, with only salal beneath the scrawny trees. Shade is minimal.

At 0.75 (1.2 km) and 2 mi (3.2 km), waterfalls are visible (at least into July) west-northwest on the north side of Davis Peak. At 1.5 mi (2.4 km) the view south is to Pyramid and Colonial peaks.

The grade briefly relents, and views open, near the national park boundary at 2.7 mi (4.3 km). The trail then traverses north into the **Sourdough Creek drainage**. Your goal is the green, alpine ridge visible above (northeast).

You might notice a left spur at 3 mi (5 km), just as the trail curves north around the ridge. It climbs 800 ft (244 m) to a viewpoint near the satellite dish above Diablo. The trail is narrow, overgrown, rarely used. Skip it. Stay on the main trail to the summit—vastly more impressive.

Views expand from 3.5 mi (5.6 km) onward. Park Creek Pass is visible southeast, up Thunder Creek valley. The trail proceeds through low brush and flowers and (through mid-July) crosses meltwater creeklets.

At 4.2 mi (6.8 km), 5000 ft (1524 m), **Sourdough Creek** is a welcome sight. Water is plentiful here. On the ridge west of the creek are treed campsites. Visible across Hwy 20 are Ruby Mtn (southeast) and Snowfield Peak (south). You're now just 1.3 mi (2.1 km) shy of and 985 ft (300 m) below the summit. Persevere.

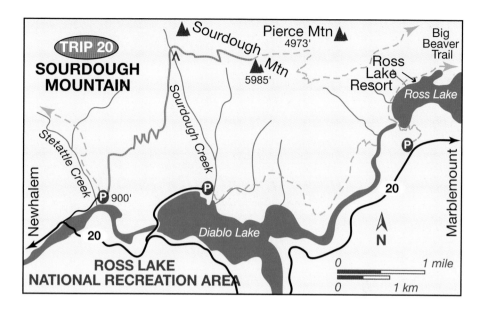

The trail resumes across the creek, just below the largest grey boulder on the left. Traverse east on alpine slopes, then enter a rocky, possibly muddy, slide area. If snow-covered, this stretch can be difficult. Beyond, ascend short switchbacks north to the summit ridge.

Upon gaining the ridge, if you encounter a snowbank (which can linger into August), don't go over it. Bear right. Stay on the southwest side of the ridge for the final 0.3 mi (0.5 km) to the fire lookout. This might still require you to negotiate snow, but the lookout is atop the actual summit of **Sourdough Mtn**, at 5.5 mi (8.9 km), 5985 ft (1824 m). That's 4777 ft (1456 m) above Diablo Lake directly below (south), and 4381 ft (1335 m) above Ross Lake (east).

The fire lookout, built in 1933, was among the first in the U.S. It's now closed to the public. The superlative vista, however, remains unchanged, and the way to enjoy it fully is with a North Cascades map in hand.

In the unlikely event that you want to hike farther, it's possible to explore northwest, cross-country, along the crest of Sourdough Mtn. The trail you followed to the summit also continues east, descending to Ross Lake (see *Green Trails* map Ross Lake 16).

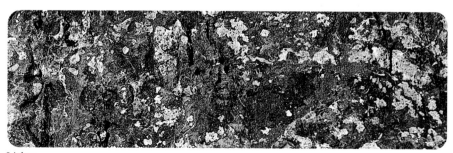

Lichen

TRIP 21
FOURTH OF JULY PASS SHOULDER SEASON

LOCATION	Ross Lake National Recreation Area
ROUND TRIP	10.6 mi (17.1 km) to pass
SHUTTLE TRIP	11.4 mi (18.3 km)
ELEVATION GAIN	2400 ft (732 m) to pass, 2880 ft (878 m) on shuttle trip
KEY ELEVATIONS	Colonial Creek trailhead 1200 ft (366 m)
	pass 3600 ft (1097 m)
	Panther Creek trailhead 1800 ft (549 m)
HIKING TIME	4½ to 5½ hours for round trip, 5 to 6 hours for shuttle trip
DIFFICULTY	moderate
MAPS	*Green Trails* Diablo Dam 48, Mt. Logan 49

OPINION

After a long, frigid winter, jump start your stone-cold-dead battery by hiking to Fourth of July Pass. The views of Neve Glacier, Colonial Peak and Snowfield Peak are jolting. And the sense of adventure you can attain here, compared to other shoulder-season options, is cathartic.

Some years, the trail is snow-free in May. But because the pass is treed and most of the trail is in forest, hike elsewhere during summer—*in* the alpine zone instead of just peering up at it.

You have options: dayhike from Thunder Creek to the pass, dayhike from Panther Creek to the pass, camp overnight at the pass, or dayhike all the way through starting at either end.

Since it's possible for robust hikers to complete the one-way journey in five or six hours, why not see it all? And why lug a full pack? If you can't arrange a car shuttle, stick out your thumb on the highway at the other end. It's a short, easy hitch.

If you choose to camp, the sites at Fourth of July Pass are superb: on a narrow shelf on the side of Ruby Mtn, with an unobstructed vista of the icy heights above.

Start on the more inviting Thunder Creek side, especially if you're just going up to the pass and back. The Panther Creek drainage is narrower and darker, and the trail is brushier. Panther is where Edgar Allen Poe would hang out; Thunder is Walt Whitman's kind of place. Both are worthwhile, but most people will feel more motivated to get out of Panther than into it, so it makes a better exit.

You'll find something to enjoy throughout the journey. Powerful yet peaceful Thunder Creek has a calming, almost hypnotic effect. The ascent to Fourth of July Pass is on a well-maintained trail, through airy, light forest. The pass itself offers a surprisingly magnificent view, so try not to stop for lunch until you get there. Panther Creek is a wild creature, snarling, roaring, slashing and ripping its way down the mountain.

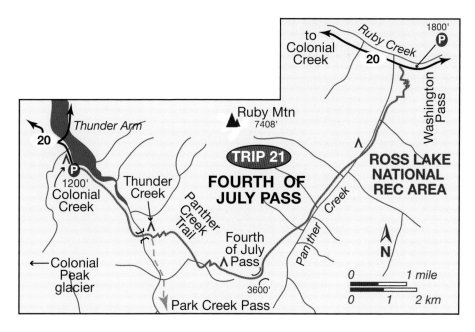

Unless the trail's been brushed, expect all manner of fanged plants to claw at your legs on the Panther Creek descent. Also be prepared for a surprise. Just when you think the highway is around the next bend, and you feel the hike down Panther Creek is over, wham: the trail climbs several hundred feet, for no apparent reason other than to wring more sweat from your brow. Don't worry. You haven't taken a wrong turn. Keep plugging uphill. The trail *does* eventually top out. It then sends you directly downhill to the highway.

FACT

BY VEHICLE

From the Diablo-townsite turnoff, drive Hwy 20 southeast 4.3 mi (6.9 km) to Colonial Creek campground on Diablo Lake. Turn southeast into the big parking lot, then proceed through the campground to the smaller parking lot at the trailhead. Elevation: 1200 ft (366 m).

To arrange a shuttle, leave your second vehicle at the East Bank trailhead on Hwy 20. It's 8.2 mi (13.2 km) east of Colonial Creek, on the north side of the highway. The Panther Creek trail intersects the south side of the highway 0.3 mi (0.5 km) west of there, at 1800 ft (549 m).

ON FOOT

The trail leads southeast, along the west shore of Diablo Lake's Thunder Arm. Ignore the signed nature trail. Proceed upstream along the west bank of Thunder Creek.

About 30 minutes from the trailhead, cross a bridge to the creek's east bank, pass **Thunder Creek camp**, and reach a signed junction at 2 mi (3.2 km). Right continues following Thunder Creek upstream generally south. Go left for Fourth of July Pass and begin a steep, switchbacking ascent generally east-northeast.

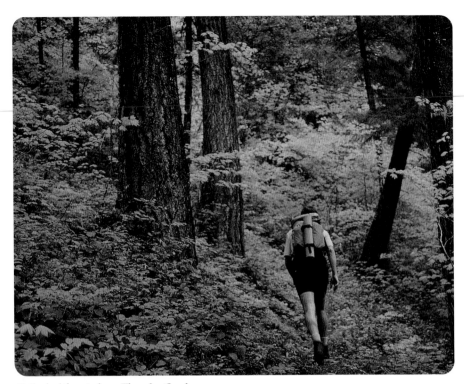

Cathedral forest along Thunder Creek

After traversing south-southeast, then switchbacking generally east again, the trail turns southeast to reach **Fourth of July camp** at 4.6 mi (7.4 km), 3500 ft (1067 m). It's left (north), above the trail, near a creeklet. Proceed east, past the tiny ponds called **Panther Potholes**. Cross broad, flat, **Fourth of July Pass** at 5.3 mi (8.5 km), 3600 ft (1097 m).

On the east side of the pass, the trail drops steeply north, then northeast to **Panther Creek**. Continuing downstream above the northwest bank, cross a few tributaries and an avalanche swath where your might encounter snow. At 8.7 mi (14 km) arrive at **Panther camp** and cross a bridge to the creek's southeast bank.

Proceed downstream (northeast) until the trail turns right and begins a startling, switchbacking ascent generally east. Gain 480 ft (146 m), then promptly lose that elevation descending north to intersect **Hwy 20** at 11.4 mi (18.3 km), 1800 ft (549 m).

When you set foot on pavement, you'll be 7.9 mi (12.7 km) east of Colonial Creek campground, and 0.3 km (0.5 mi) west of the East Bank trailhead.

TRIP 22
EASY PASS

LOCATION	North Cascades National Park
ROUND TRIP	7.2 mi (11.6 km)
ELEVATION GAIN	2800 ft (853 m)
KEY ELEVATIONS	trailhead 3700 ft (1128 m), pass 6500 ft (1981 m)
HIKING TIME	3½ to 4½ hours
DIFFICULTY	moderate
MAP	*Green Trails* Mt. Logan 49

OPINION

The miners who clambered over the North Cascades were powerful, obstinate brutes. What most of us today would consider impenetrable or insurmountable, they looked upon as entirely feasible. So when they named this cleft "Easy Pass," they were appraising the challenge it posed relative to other, far more laborious passages.

What was easy for a turn-of-the-century miner might not be easy for you. But the lavish scenic reward at the pass will justify your effort to get there no matter how it rates on your personal difficulty scale. And if you're strong, you certainly won't consider this an overly strenuous hike.

In about one hour, you'll be surging into the subalpine zone, enjoying expansive views. Near the pass, a great cliff towers above the trail, perhaps sharpening your sense of impending drama. And the scene you'll witness from the pass is dramatic indeed.

The principal sights are, from east to west, Fisher Peak, Black Peak behind and above it, and Mt. Arriva. West-southwest is Mt. Logan. Far west, above Thunder Creek Valley, is Tricouni Peak and glacier-clad Klawatti Peak. Neve Glacier is northwest.

For the optimal vantage, continue through the pass. Just before descending, find a seat on the heather slope, high above the emerald depths of Fisher Basin, and marvel at the magnitude of the wilderness beyond. A short scramble above either side of the pass will further improve your perspective.

Easy Pass cleaves Ragged Ridge in a west-east swath. Heavily shaded by the ridge, the pass tends to hold snow well into summer. You'll be lucky if it's safe to hike without an ice axe by mid-July. It's usually inaccessible to hikers until August. If you arrive when the final 0.2 mi (0.3 km) of trail below the pass is still snow-covered, bare rock to the right might help you safely attain your goal.

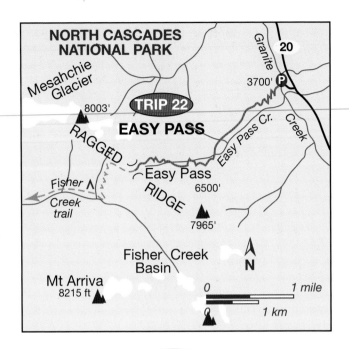

BY VEHICLE

Drive Hwy 20 southeast 21.5 mi (34.6 km) from Colonial Creek campground on Diablo Lake, or northwest 6.3 mi (10.1 km) from Rainy Pass. Turn west onto a short spur to reach the trailhead parking lot at 3700 ft (1128 m).

ON FOOT

Heading south, the trail delivers you to a bridged crossing of **Granite Creek** in 0.2 mi (0.3 km). Beyond the far bank begin a switchbacking ascent generally southwest through a forest of western hemlock and Pacific silver fir.

At 2 mi (3.2 km), cross a footlog spanning **Easy Pass Creek**. The grade steepens, heading generally west. Surmount treeline near 2.3 mi (3.7 km) and cross the creek thrice more—rockhopping or on footlogs.

The notch of Easy Pass is now visible ahead (west). East, across the valley, are the rugged spires of Mt. Hardy. Cutthroat Peak is southeast.

Approaching the pass, the trail switchbacks up the right (north) side of the gully. The final 0.5 mi (0.8 km) is through heather and berry bushes, then talus. After crossing the signed national-park boundary, enter 6500-ft (1981-m) **Easy Pass** at 3.6 mi (5.8 km).

Larch, alpine fir, mountain hemlock and whitebark pine adorn the pass, which bisects Ragged Ridge. Enhance your view by scrambling higher—either north-northwest or southeast.

Camping is prohibited at the pass. Backpackers must proceed west, descending 2.1 mi (3.4 km) to a no-fire campsite at 5200 ft (1585 m) in Fisher Basin. From there, continuing east along the Fisher Creek trail is a long, viewless slog. Better to enjoy Easy Pass as a dayhike.

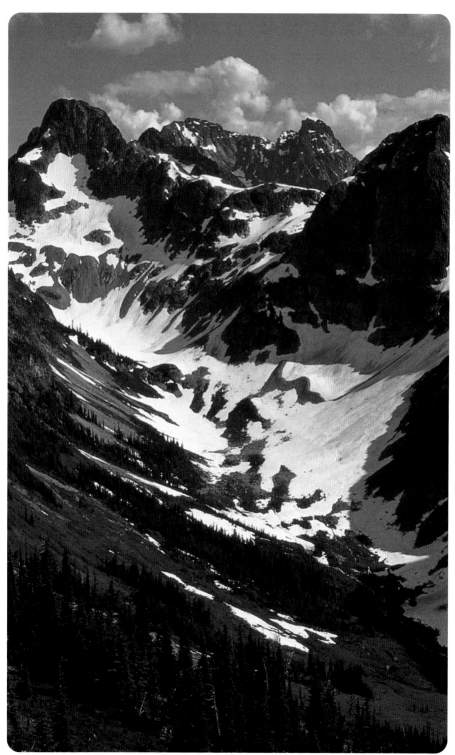

Fisher Basin, Fisher Peak, and Black Peak, from Easy Pass

TRIP 23

HEATHER PASS / MAPLE PASS

LOCATION	North Cascades Scenic Hwy Area
LOOP	7.2 mi (11.6 km) including Lake Ann excursion
ELEVATION GAIN	1995 ft (608 m)
KEY ELEVATIONS	trailhead 4855 ft (1480 m), Heather Pass 6100 ft (1859 m)
	Maple Pass 6600 ft (2012 m), highpoint 6850 ft (2088 m)
HIKING TIME	3½ to 4½ hours
DIFFICULTY	easy
MAPS	*Green Trails* Mt. Logan 49, Washington Pass 50

OPINION

Spud life—couch, beer, potato chips, televised sports—is a pillar of American culture. Be glad of it. If Americans were a predominantly vigorous, adventurous lot, you'd have to make reservations for dayhikes to spectacular vantage points like these.

Heather and Maple passes are already crowded enough, for good reason: few hikes anywhere are so instantly gratifying. The trail flings you into the alpine zone. You'll see waterfalls, flowery meadows, two majestic lake cirques, and craggy peaks, all within a few hours. Plus this is a loop.

Here you can fully appreciate the contrast between the two sides of the Pacific Crest. To the east are dry, brown, stark, rocky peaks above sparse forest. To the west are lush, green slopes and glacier-capped mountains above big timber. The view changes radically when you swivel your head: from the yellow and rusty scree slopes along the PCT between Cutthroat and Granite passes, to the abundant greenery ringing the snowcone of Glacier Peak.

Though short, this trip is a series of scenic crescendos. But getting beyond the first one, Lake Ann, can be difficult on a sunny day. After admiring the tremendous cirque, some people end the hike right there. They find a smooth log, stretch out and doze, lulled by the music of the cascade at the far shore. Resist temptation. Push on. Soon you'll be striding atop the green slopes hugging Lake Ann. Great mountains will swirl about you. Then comes the exciting plunge beside the Rainy Lake cirque. Along the way, you'll often have the pleasure of seeing far ahead to the trail you'll be walking, or way back where you came from.

Come here midweek when there's less traffic on the trail and the highway. On a typical weekend, you'll hear cars whizzing past the trailhead for the first 20 minutes and last 40 minutes of your hike. You can also escape the crowd by rambling the sketchy-but-easy-to-follow route from Heather Pass to Lewis Lake and on to Wing Lake beneath Black Peak.

Do the loop counter-clockwise. Go to Lake Ann and Heather Pass first, then drop to Rainy Lake from Maple Pass. It would be exhausting and

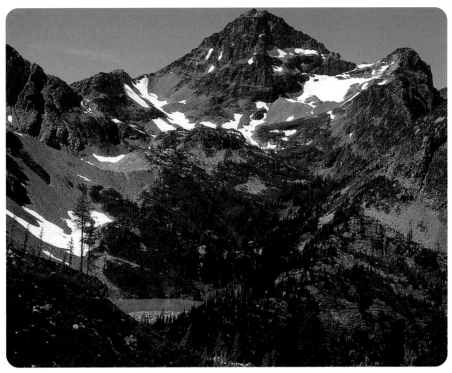

Lewis Lake, from Heather Pass

discouraging to ascend above Rainy Lake first. But beware: it's a cartilage cruncher coming down. Though this descent is not shown on some maps, the trail is signed and obvious.

FACT

BY VEHICLE

Drive Hwy 20 to Rainy Pass. It's 37.2 mi (60 km) southeast of Newhalem, or 20.8 mi (33.5 km) southwest of Early Winters. From either approach, turn west into the Rainy Pass picnic-area parking lot, at 4855 ft (1480 m).

ON FOOT

The trail departs the south end of the parking lot, near where you entered. Follow the steep, dirt path. The level, paved walkway will be your return route from Rainy Lake.

The trail gains 670 ft (204 m) in the first 1 mi (0.6 km), switchbacking through open forest, soon heading generally south-southwest. Visible across the highway are Cutthroat Peak (northeast) and Whistler Mtn (east). From meadowy slopes, attain a view into the Lake Ann cirque and of Frisco Mtn to the south. At 1.2 mi (1.9 km) the trail turns west into the narrow valley cleaved by Lake Ann's outlet stream.

At 1.3 mi (2.1 km), 5400 ft (1646 m), reach a signed fork. Left leads 0.5 mi (0.8 km) west-southwest through subalpine forest and marshy meadows to

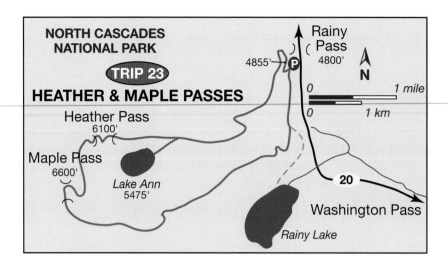

Lake Ann. Look for trumpet shaped, pink monkeyflower, orange and yellow columbines, and subalpine spirea, which has small, pink blossoms in a flat cluster at the top. Camping is prohibited here.

From the 1.3-mi (2.1-km) fork, the main trail goes right. Ascend a rockslide with open views of Lake Ann below. Heading generally west, reach 6100-ft (1859-m) **Heather Pass** at 2.25 mi (3.6 km).

Just before the pass, a right fork descends through heather. It leads to Lewis Lake at 5702 ft (1738 m) and continues to Wing Lake at 6905 ft (2105 m). Both lakes are visible from a switchback just above the pass. Lewis is nearby west-northwest. Wing is beyond, in the cirque beneath 8970-ft (2734-m) Black Peak.

From Heather Pass the trail ascends 260 ft (79 m) toward Corteo Peak. Copper Pass and Stiletto Peak are visible east and slightly south. The trail contours south from Heather Pass 0.5 mi (0.8 km), then ascends 240 ft (73 m) to Maple Pass. Visible from the ridge are Corteo Peak (nearby west), Storm King Mtn (distant, slightly south of west), and Mt. Benzarino (southwest).

Reach 6600-ft (2012-m) **Maple Pass** at 3.1 mi (5 km). Maple Creek valley is deep below. Glacier Peak is visible southwest, across Glacier Peak Wilderness.

To complete the loop, curve east along the ridgecrest, topping out on a 6850-ft (2088-m) shoulder of Frisco Mtn. Rainy Lake is 2050 ft (625 m) below. Tight, steep switchbacks descend the alpine ridge separating the Lake Ann and Rainy Lake cirques.

Near 4.5 mi (7.2 km), a hanging basin above Rainy Lake and a long waterfall tumbling into it are visible. Near 6400 ft (1951 m) the persistent switchbacks drop below treeline. The remaining descent is northeast along the ridge through viewless forest.

Reach the **paved walkway** at 5.8 mi (9.3 km). Right leads 0.6 mi (1 km) south to Rainy Lake. Go left (north) 0.4 mi (0.6 km) to reach the parking lot and complete the 6.2-mi (10-km) loop. Total distance including the 1-mi (1.6-km) Lake Ann excursion: 7.2 mi (11.6 km).

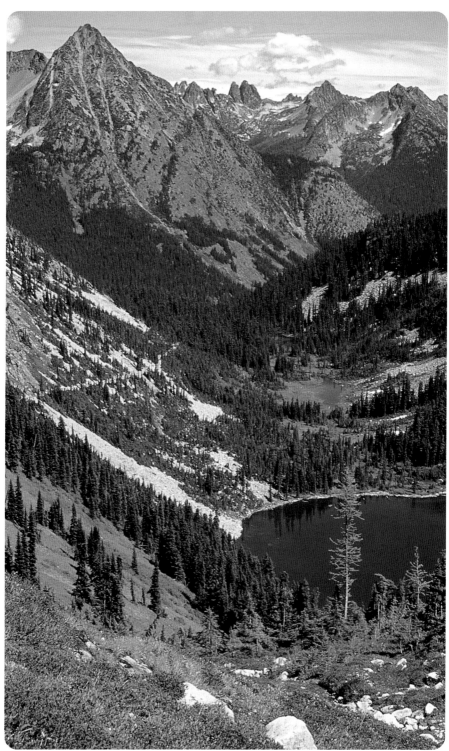

Lake Ann, from Heather Pass

TRIP 24

CUTTHROAT PASS

LOCATION	~~North Cascades Scenic Hwy Area~~ Okanogan National Forest
ROUND TRIP	10 mi (16.1 km)
ELEVATION GAIN	2000 ft (610 m)
KEY ELEVATIONS	trailhead 4800 ft (1463 m), pass 6800 ft (2073 m)
HIKING TIME	4 to 5 hours
DIFFICULTY	easy
MAP	*Green Trails* Washington Pass 50

OPINION

The Pacific Crest Trail's gentle grade enables you to maintain momentum on this easy ascent past treeline to Cutthroat Pass. Instead of hammering away with head down, you can stride—arms loose, hips swinging—and appreciate the cool forest, heather meadows and rock gardens en route. Compared to many North Cascades' trails—especially the old miners' routes that go ballistic if not vertical—such a tame path is a luxurious indulgence.

Cutthroat Pass affords sweeping views across dry-bones country: high, arid, bleak. But the jagged skyline is a spectacle nonetheless. Huge, flat, lounge-lizard boulders await you at the pass. But don't linger. Ridges on either side invite exploration. And the PCT beckons. Keep going to the knoll above Granite Pass to look down into Swamp Creek valley and out at soaring mountains.

Start this hike at Rainy Pass, as described here, rather than at Cutthroat Creek. From Rainy, the grade is gentler because it's the PCT. You'll exit the forest sooner. And your round-trip distance will be a mile shorter. Also, don't bother arranging a shuttle for a one-way trip exiting via Cutthroat Creek. You'll see Cutthroat Lake from Cutthroat Pass. Besides, the forest and meadows between Rainy and Cutthroat passes are worth seeing twice.

FACT

BY VEHICLE

Drive Hwy 20 southeast 37.2 mi (60 km) from Newhalem, or southwest 20.8 mi (33.5 km) from Early Winters. Ignore the picnic area (west). Turn east into the Rainy Pass trailhead parking lot, at 4800 ft (1463 m).

ON FOOT

Follow the Pacific Crest Trail north, initially paralleling the highway, then curving northeast up the **Porcupine Creek** drainage.

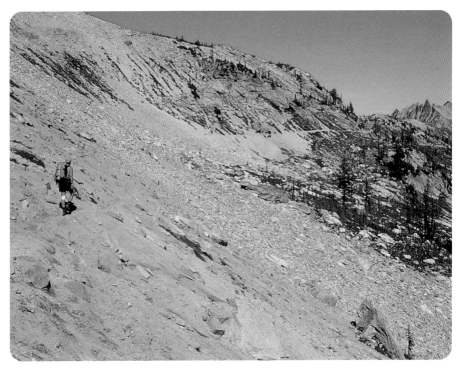

Nearing Cutthroat Pass

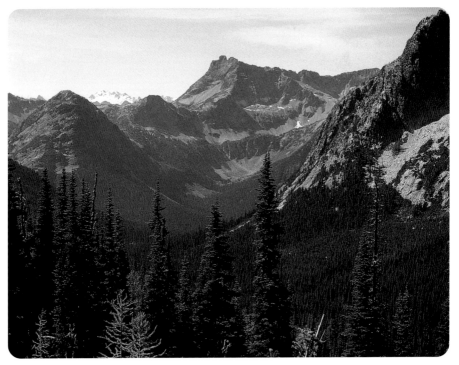

Looking southwest from Cutthroat Pass

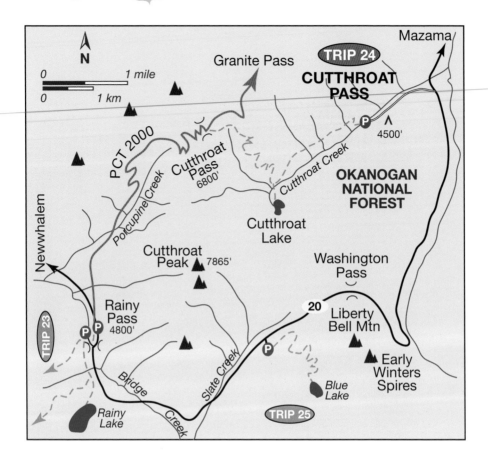

At 2 mi (3.2 km) Cutthroat Pass is visible northeast. After walking through verdant forest for 3 mi (4.8 km), enter heather meadows among sparser trees. Pass a campsite at 4 mi (6.4 km). The last 1 mi (1.6 km) is in open, rocky, alpine terrain.

Enter 6800-ft (2073-m) **Cutthroat Pass** at 5 mi (8 km). Be sure to detour south up the ridge for a superior view of nearby 7865-ft (2397-m) Cutthroat Peak (southeast) and Liberty Bell Mtn beyond it.

The PCT resumes, of course, contouring northeast on barren slopes above Cutthroat Creek canyon. A knoll at 6.4 mi (10.3 km), above where the trail switchbacks down to **Granite Pass**, allows you to survey Swamp Creek valley (northwest) and inspect Tower Mtn and Golden Horn (north-northwest).

BLUE LAKE

LOCATION	North Cascades Scenic Hwy Area
ROUND TRIP	4.4 mi (7.1 km)
ELEVATION GAIN	1100 ft (335 m)
KEY ELEVATIONS	trailhead 5200 ft (1585 m), lake 6300 ft (1920 m)
HIKING TIME	2 hours
DIFFICULTY	easy
MAP	*Green Trails* Washington Pass 50

OPINION

Beneath soaring, rose-colored cirque walls, Blue Lake is a startling deep turquoise. The Early Winters Spires are visible above—close enough for you to see the crack that earned Liberty Bell Mtn its name. The surrounding ridges are bearded with alpine larch that turn brilliant gold in fall, cranking the lake's scenic wattage even higher.

Short hikes in the North Cascades are rarely so rewarding. So Blue Lake is an optimal destination for hikers of all ages and abilities. The ascent is mild, the switchbacks long and gentle. Even if you're just driving through the park, stop here, stretch your legs, and gain a deeper appreciation for the mountains.

FACT

BY VEHICLE

Drive Hwy 20 southwest 0.8 mi (1.3 km) from Washington Pass, or east 4.2 mi (6.8 km) from Rainy Pass. Turn east into the trailhead parking area at 5200 ft (1585 m).

ON FOOT

Starting behind the outhouse, follow the trail northeast through spruce forest. It parallels the highway for 0.6 mi (1 km), so car noise is audible. Long switchbacks then begin ascending generally southeast.

At 1.5 mi (2.4 km), in a flowery avalanche meadow fed by cascading

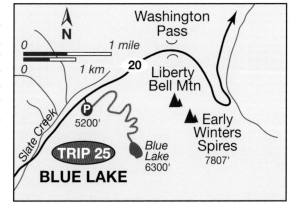

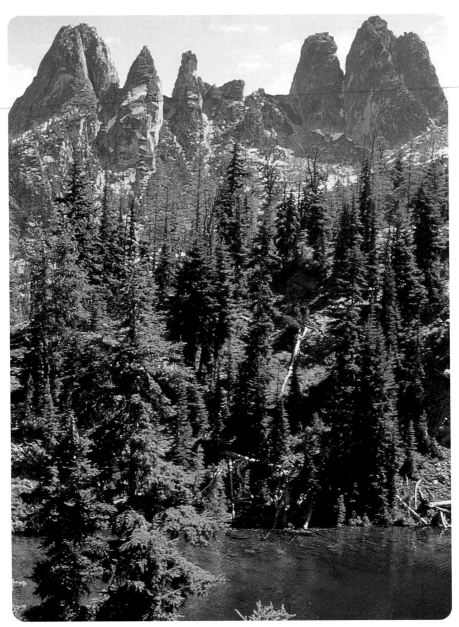

Blue Lake and the Early Winters Spires

creeks, attain views west and north. Ignore the climbers' route forking left (east) to the Early Winters Spires. Stay on the main trail: curving right (southwest) and leveling.

Rockhop the outlet stream to reach the north shore of **Blue Lake** at 2.2 mi (3.5 km), 6300 ft (1920 m). The trees are mostly larches and hardy whitebark pines. Camping is forbidden at this popular, fragile area.

WINDY PASS

LOCATION	Okanogan National Forest
ROUND TRIP	7.4 mi (11.9 km)
ELEVATION GAIN	300 ft (91 m) to, plus 700 ft (213 m) from
KEY ELEVATIONS	trailhead 6800 ft (2073 m), pass 6300 ft (1920 m)
HIKING TIME	3 to 4 hours
DIFFICULTY	easy
MAPS	*Green Trails* Washington Pass 50, Pasayten Peak 18 Jack Mtn 17 (shows route north of Woody Pass)

OPINION

The Pacific Crest Trail between Harts Pass and Windy Pass is baby-carriage gentle. It contours meadowy slopes, high above forested valleys. Views are constant—just turn your head.

Many thru-hikers cite this stretch as the easiest and most scenic of their 500-mi (805-km) trek across Washington. If you're a spirited strider, dayhiking here poses only one challenge: reining yourself in and turning around.

The Three Fools Peak massif is visible north. Glacier-headed Jack Mtn is west. Tower Mtn and Golden Horn are south. And that's but a fraction of what you'll see. If you can spare a second day in the area, dayhike to Grasshopper Pass, where you can appreciate at closer range two of the panorama's dominant features: Mt. Ballard and Azurite Peak.

Families with small children, or anyone who prefers strolling to straining, will find Windy Pass an ideal outing. The larch-strewn meadows at the pass are an easy-but-lovely destination for backpackers unwilling or unable to invest a long day on a rough trail to experience mountain glory. If you back-pack, expect chilly nights up here and possibly snow as early as September.

Although the views from the trail are excellent, the nearby fire lookout atop 7440-ft (2268-m) Slate Peak is a higher, more commanding vantage. Don't miss it. Drive the short distance to the end of the gated road, then walk 0.25 mi (0.4 km) to the summit. Ideally, come here after your Windy Pass hike. Watch the sun set on a sweeping North Cascades panorama, including distant Mt. Baker.

Before traipsing farther north on the PCT, ponder the effort/reward ratio. Past the 6700-ft (2042-m) ridgecrest just beyond Windy Pass, the trail is above treeline for only a short spurt along Devils Backbone and for about 6 mi (10 km) between Goat Lakes and the north end of spectacular Lakeview Ridge. Looking west from the high, open slopes of Three Fools Peak, you'll see stalwart mountains in the distance. Then you'll be in forest most of the 17.7 mi (28.5 km) to the northern terminus of the PCT on Canada's Hwy 3. There's also the logistical challenge of arranging return transportation from

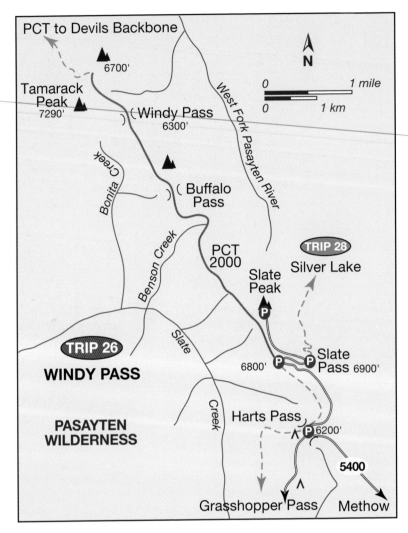

Manning Provincial Park to Harts Pass. Unless you have a willing shuttle-slave, it's a complex ordeal requiring public transport and hitchhiking.

Some years, the Windy Pass trailhead isn't accessible until mid-August. Check with the Winthrop Ranger District about road and trail conditions. It's best to come here in September, when the days are cool and dreamy.

FACT

BY VEHICLE

Drive Hwy 20 northwest 13.2 mi (21.2 km) from Winthrop, or southeast 1.5 mi (2.4 km) from Early Winters. At the sign for Mazama, turn northeast, cross the Methow River bridge, then turn left at the T-junction onto Harts Pass Road. Proceed 9.1 mi (14.6 km) northwest to a junction. Turn right and continue another 10 mi (16.1 km) to Harts Pass at 6200 ft (1890 m). Bear right onto

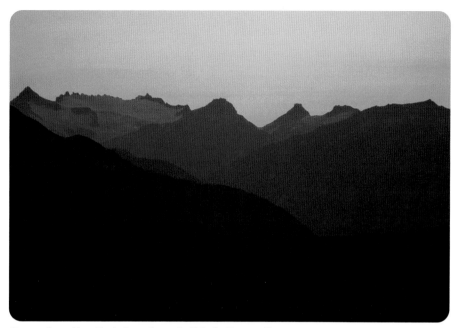

Sunset from Slate Peak, just above the Windy Pass trail

Slate Peak Road 600 and drive 1.5 mi (2.4 km) northwest to the first switch-back (pointing west), where there's a small, trailhead parking area at 6800 ft (2073 m).

ON FOOT

Initially heading northeast, this section of the PCT begins by gently climb-ing a bench. It then contours generally northwest around Slate Peak, eases into Benson Basin, rises to Buffalo Pass, descends above Barron Basin and Bonita Creek, and at 3.7 mi (6 km) reaches the meadows and campsites of 6300-ft (1920-m) **Windy Pass**.

For more views, continue northwest. Pass campsites and a reliable water source in a basin at 4.1 mi (6.6 km). The trail switchbacks up to reach a ridge-crest at 4.4 mi (7.1 km), 6700 ft (2042 m). This is a good place for dayhikers to turn around.

Continuing north, the PCT descends to Foggy Pass at 6 mi (10 km), 6200 ft (1890 m). From the northeast ridge of Devils Backbone, at 8.25 mi (13.3 km), it drops into trees and reaches 5100-ft (1554-m), forested Holman Pass at 13.2 mi (21.2 km). Near 15 mi (24.1 km) reach the meadowy Goat Lakes basin beneath Holman Peak by veering off-trail 0.5 mi (0.8 km) east. Near Woody Pass, 18.4 mi (29.6 km) from Slate Peak Road, begin the long, high contour beneath Three Fools Peak and along Lakeview Ridge. Near 21.5 mi (34.6 km) the PCT drops off the crest and, for most of the remaining 17.7 mi (28.5 km) to Hwy 3 in Canada's Manning Provincial Park, is in deep forest.

GRASSHOPPER PASS

LOCATION	Okanogan National Forest
ROUND TRIP	11 mi (17.7 km)
ELEVATION GAIN	1000 ft (305 m) to, plus 1000 ft (305 m) from
KEY ELEVATIONS	trailhead 6400 ft (1951 m), pass 6750 ft (2057 m) highpoint 7125 ft (2172 m)
HIKING TIME	4 to 5½ hours
DIFFICULTY	easy
MAP	*Green Trails* Washington Pass 50

OPINION

Alpine scenery attained with little effort, and a likelihood of sunny skies make the trip to Grasshopper Pass a welcome change from the steeper trails and wetter climate farther west. It's one of those rare sections of the Pacific Crest Trail where, starting at a high-elevation trailhead, you can blithely enjoy what long-distance trekkers struggle to reach.

You leave the trees at the trailhead, so views are constant. Typical of the eastern Cascades, the landscape resembles the drier, more sparsely vegetated Front Range of Colorado, or even the high deserts of Arizona. The route is a long, snaking contour of rocky slopes.

After rounding the first peak, you can look across a big horseshoe bend and see the path you'll follow to the pass, so there's no element of surprise. Still, the trail is a joy to walk. The Pasayten Wilderness stretches northeast across the horizon. Nearby are Azurite Peak (southwest) and Mt. Ballard (northwest).

This hike is more dramatic than the one to Windy Pass, just north of Harts Pass. Both trails afford expansive vistas, but this one is closer to jagged peaks and in places has steep dropoffs on both sides.

Some years, the trailhead isn't accessible until mid-August. Check with the Winthrop Ranger District about road and trail conditions. It's best to come here in September, when the days are cool and dreamy, and when you won't be searching for shade—because there isn't any.

FACT

BY VEHICLE

Drive Hwy 20 northwest 13.2 mi (21.2 km) from Winthrop, or southeast 1.5 mi (2.4 km) from Early Winters. At the sign for Mazama, turn northeast, cross the Methow River bridge, then turn left at the T-junction onto Harts Pass Road. Proceed 9.1 mi (14.6 km) northwest to a junction. Turn right and continue another 10 mi (16.1 km) to Harts Pass at 6200 ft (1890 m). Turn left at the pass, following the sign for Meadows campground. Reach road's end and the trailhead parking area in 2 mi (3.2 km), at 6400 ft (1951 m).

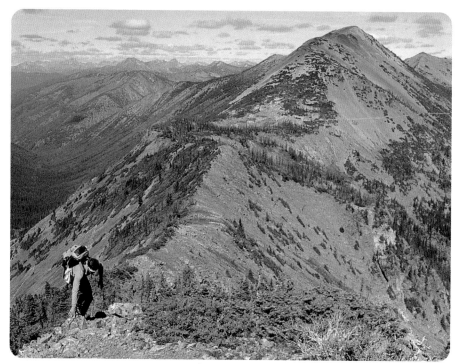

Topping-out on knob south of Grasshopper Pass

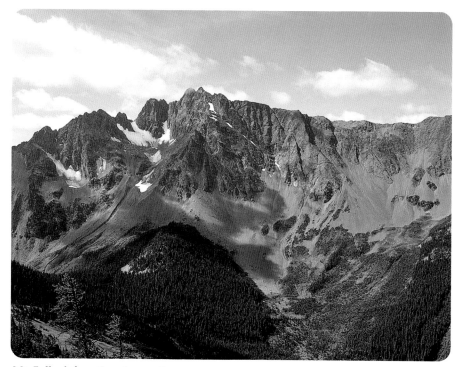

Mt. Ballard, from Grasshopper Pass

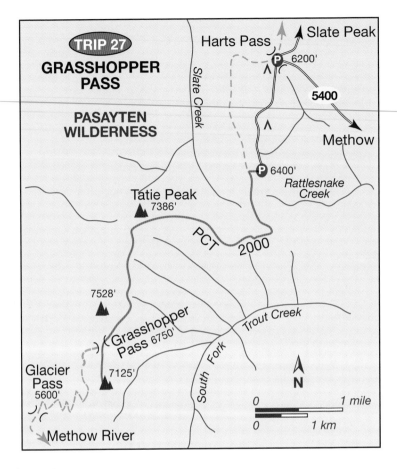

ON FOOT

One minute beyond the trailhead, reach a T-junction with the Pacific Crest Trail. Go left (south) contouring along an east-facing slope.

The trail soon curves right (west) onto a south-facing slope—beneath an unnamed 7405-ft (2257-m) peak—to a saddle above the headwaters of Slate Creek in Ninetynine Basin (north).

Continue west under 7386-ft (2251-m) **Tatie Peak**, to a 6880-ft (2097-m) saddle on its southwest slope. Directly west is 8301-ft (2530-m) Mt. Ballard. The trail then turns south and descends into a basin, reaching a campsite and dependable creek at 3.8 mi (6.1 km), 6640 ft (2024 m).

Ascend south-southwest to **Grasshopper Pass**—a small saddle at 5 mi (8 km), 6750 ft (2057 m). Beyond, the PCT descends steeply west to 5600-ft (1707-m) Glacier Pass. Azurite Peak is west-southwest.

Improve your view significantly by turning left, off the trail, just before the plunging switchbacks. Follow a bootbeaten route south along the ridgeline. Fifteen minutes of upward effort will put you atop a 7125-ft (2172 m) knob at 5.5 mi (8.9 km), where the southern panorama is complete.

Competent scramblers can leave the trail to Grasshopper Pass almost anywhere en route and ascend one or more of the small peaks above. It's even possible to negotiate the entire crest between the trailhead and the pass.

SILVER LAKE

LOCATION	Pasayten Wilderness
ROUND TRIP	9.2 mi (14.8 km)
ELEVATION GAIN	1800 ft (549 m) to lake and back
KEY ELEVATIONS	trailhead 6900 ft (2104 m), lake 6256 ft (1907 m)
HIKING TIME	4 to 5 hours
DIFFICULTY	easy
MAPS	*Green Trails* Washington Pass 50, Pasayten Peak 18

OPINION

The cathedral forests of the North Cascades are awe-inspiring. But even tree huggers enjoy an occasional reprieve from the dark, valley-bottom groves. Here's where to come up for air.

The road climbs all the way to a mountaintop fire lookout. You start hiking in the alpine zone. You ascend only gradually, mostly on the return. You dip into the subalpine zone only briefly.

What's more, you can car camp up here and hike other trails that offer equally easy, scenic, high-elevation cruising. One leads to Windy Pass. Another to Grasshopper Pass.

If there's anything to criticize about this trip, it's the destination. Silver Lake is not spectacular. It's small, cloaked in forest, tucked into an obscure hollow below Pasayten Peak. It's merely a demarcation. "Turn around here," it says to dayhikers.

The climax is actually near the trailhead, at the fire-lookout site, where the view encompasses the bulk of the North Cascades (west), the Pasayten Wilderness (north and east), and the peaks girding Rainy and Washington passes (south).

But between the trailhead and Silver Lake, the trail affords blissful striding. It sidles along Gold Ridge, through meadows flecked with larch and silver fir, across creeklets slithering off the ridgecrest. Below is the Middle Fork Pasayten River valley. Above and beyond are Devils Peak and Wildcat Mtn.

Bring your little hikers-in-training. Within a half-mile you'll enter a huge, lush meadow where you can contentedly sit and gaze while the kids do their tripped-out biologist routine. In summer, the wildflower show is loud. In fall, the golden larch are plugged in and turned on.

You've got plenty of kid-like curiosity and energy yourself? Create a circuit by hiking the trail north to Silver Lake, then ascending to the crest of Gold Ridge and following it back, rejoining the path for the final 2 mi (3.2 km) to the trailhead.

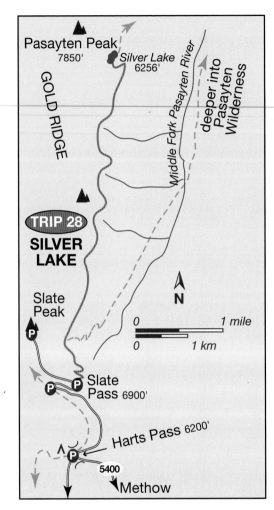

Pasayten Peak
7850'

GOLD RIDGE

Silver Lake
6256'

Middle Fork Pasayten River

deeper into
Pasayten
Wilderness

TRIP 28
**SILVER
LAKE**

Slate
Peak
Ⓟ

N

0 _____ 1 mile
0 _____ 1 km

Ⓟ Ⓟ Slate
Pass 6900'

Harts Pass 6200'

5400
Ⓟ

Methow

FACT

BY VEHICLE

Drive Hwy 20 northwest 13.2 mi (21.2 km) from Winthrop, or southeast 1.5 mi (2.4 km) from Early Winters. At the sign for Mazama, turn northeast, cross the Methow River bridge, then turn left at the T-junction onto Harts Pass Road. Proceed 9.1 mi (14.6 km) northwest to a junction. Turn right and continue another 10 mi (16.1 km) to Harts Pass at 6200 ft (1890 m). Bear right onto Slate Peak Road 600 and drive northwest. At 11.5 mi (18.5 km) switchback beyond the Windy Pass trailhead. At 11.8 mi (19 km) reach the next switchback (pointing east) and the Slate Pass trailhead. Park on the southeast side of the road, at 6900 (2104 m).

ON FOOT

Heading northwest, the trail ascends 80 ft (24 m) to a ridge. It then gradually descends north into a meadowy basin decorated with larch.

Your destination, Silver Lake, is directly north of the trailhead, and that will remain your general direction of travel.

In 15 minutes, at 0.4 mi (0.6 km), 6800 ft (2073 m), proceed north on the main trail. Ignore the faint, unsigned, right fork: trail 478A descending southeast, eventually intersecting the Robinson Creek trail.

Reach a junction at 1.3 mi (2.1 km), 6500 ft (1981 m). Go left (northeast), skirting Haystack Mtn, and continuing north along the east side of Gold Ridge. Right descends steeply east-southeast then follows the Middle Fork Pasayten River north.

The trail stays near 6800 ft (2073 m) for the next 1.5 mi (2.4 km) through meadows and among larch and silver fir, with only minor ups and downs. The forested Middle Fork Pasayten River valley is 1500 ft (457 m) below.

After descending through beautiful spruce forest, enter another stand of larch and cross two creek drainages. About an hour from the trailhead, pass a grand larch tree 1.5 yd/m in diameter.

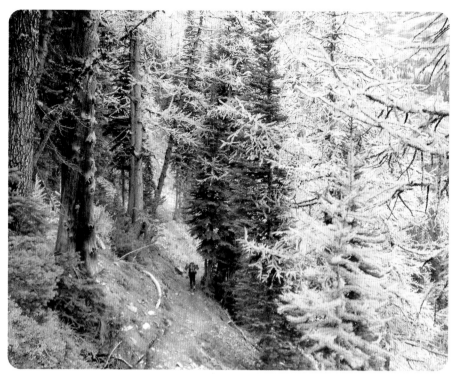

Alpine larch are profuse along the Silver Lake trail.

Cross a third stream about 1¼ hours from the trailhead. A short, steep ascent then crests a **shoulder** of Gold Ridge at 6720 ft (2048 m). Having now hiked about 1¾ hours, you're above a small, forested basin. The trail plunges into it, reaching the northeast shore of **Silver Lake** at 4.6 mi (7.4 km), 6256 ft (1907 m).

Unless you're camping at the lake, you can spare yourself the elevation loss. Go right, off trail, to glimpse the lake from atop the shoulder. Beyond the the lake, the trail continues north-northeast, crosses Silver Creek 1 mi (1.6 km) farther, then ascends to Buckskin Ridge.

Where the trail crosses the shoulder en route to Silver Lake, scramblers can ascend cross-country (southwest, then west) to the crest of **Gold Ridge**. From there, it's possible to follow the crest south, topping out at 7456 ft (2273 m), then descending south to intersect the trail about 2 mi (3.2 km) north of the trailhead.

The ridgecrest panorama includes 7850-ft (2393-m) Pasayten Peak (nearby north), 8096-ft (2468-m) Mt. Rolo (northwest), 8557-ft (2618-m) Osceola Peak (farther northwest), the Methow River Valley (southeast), and the craggy peaks above Washington Pass (south).

TRIP 29

HIDDEN LAKE PEAKS LOOKOUT

LOCATION	Mt. Baker-Snoqualmie National Forest
	North Cascades National Park
ROUND TRIP	9 mi (14.5 km)
ELEVATION GAIN	3200 ft (975 m)
KEY ELEVATIONS	trailhead 3700 ft (1128 m), lookout 6900 ft (2103 m)
HIKING TIME	4½ to 6 hours
DIFFICULTY	moderate
MAPS	*Green Trails* Marblemount 47 (shows Roads 15 and 1540) Diablo Dam 48, Cascade Pass 80

OPINION

It's a dispiriting fact that most people who hike—even those who consider themselves keen hikers—spend only a tiny fraction of each summer on the trail. Their hiking "lives" are more fantasy than reality. So when they daydream about hiking, they imagine themselves on trails like this one: the kind that will fuel their ardor through long periods of abstinence; the kind that prove the North Cascades truly are the American Alps.

Well before the summit, you'll traverse meadows and boulder fields that would themselves be a satisfying destination if the trail didn't continue. Be grateful it does. Of all the hiker-accessible lookouts in the North Cascades, only Sourdough Mtn offers a view as impressive as this one above Hidden Lake. You can see east over the Stehekin Valley, west to the ocean, north to Mt. Baker, south to Mt. Rainier. Most of the great mountains of the range are visible from this apex. You're surrounded by serrated ridges, spiky peaks, alpine slopes, steep couloirs, and hanging valleys. Though easy to ignore amid the overwhelming beauty, you can also see ugly clearcuts west and south. It is, after all, a former logging road that whisks you to the trailhead.

Don't hike here on a rainy or even cloudy day; you need a blue sky to fully appreciate the 360° vista. Also keep in mind that the trail's upper reaches can remain snow-covered well into summer. Before setting out, check with the National Park Wilderness Info Center in Marblemount.

The lookout cabin is open to the public. It sleeps four. If you hope to spend the night there, it's first come, first served, so bring a tent in case it's occupied. You'll find campsites 400 ft (122 m) below the notch, on the way to Hidden Lake. There are more near the lake's east end, where the ground is flatter. Pick your way over talus to the lakeshore.

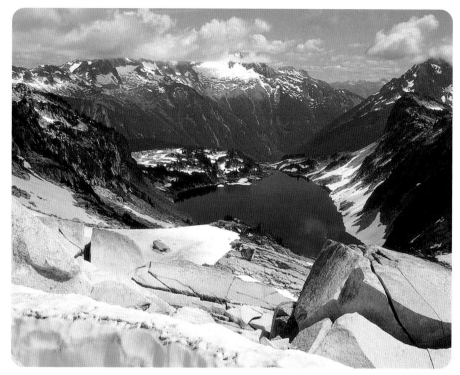

Hidden Lake, from near Hidden Lake Peaks lookout

FACT

BY VEHICLE

At the east edge of Marblemount, where Hwy 20 bends north, go straight (east) onto Cascade River Road and immediately cross the Skagit River. At 0.7 mi (1.1 km) pass the Rockport-Cascade Road on the right. Continue east on Cascade River Road 15. Pavement ends at 5.2 mi (8.4 km). At 8.3 mi (13.4 km), pass the entrance to Marble Creek campground. At 9.8 mi (15.8 km), turn left (east) onto Road 1540. It's steep and narrow, with a treacherous dropoff the final 0.3 mi (0.5 km). (A jeep departing the trailhead tumbled off the edge here because the driver didn't stop for an ascending vehicle. Be cautious.) At 14.6 mi (23.5 km), 3700 ft (1128 m), arrive at the trailhead. The parking lot is narrow, so turn around before you park. Don't block the turnaround area near the trailhead sign at road's end.

ON FOOT

The first 0.25 mi (0.4 km) east is through brush and over creeklets. Then walk in deep forest northeast for 0.75 mi (1.2 km) on moderate switchbacks. At 1 mi (1.6 km) cross **East Fork Sibley Creek** and burst into meadows dappled with alder, cow parsnip, Indian hellebore, penstemon, monkeypod, tiger lilies, thistle, paintbrush and bluebells. There are waterfalls above.

The trail ascends east as it traverses to the head of the East Fork. The narrow path is on steeply slanted grass-and-dirt slopes that can be muddy and

TRIP 29

HIDDEN LAKE PEAKS LOOKOUT

Marblemount

1540

Sibley Creek

MT. BAKER-SNOQUALMIE NATIONAL FOREST

15

P 3700'

The Triad 6804'

Hidden Lake Peaks

Hidden Lake 5733'

N

0   1 mile
0   1 km

Cascade Pass trailhead

lookout 6900'

Johannesburg Mtn

slick. Heavy rain has previously washed out this section of trail. Check with the National Park Wilderness Info Center in Marblemount about the latest conditions.

At 1.7 mi (2.7 km) you can look from meadows across to the rocky course the trail follows on a northwest-facing slope. Cross the creek at 2.2 mi (3.5 km). The rich meadowland changes to predominantly alpine heather as the terrain gets rockier. At 2.3 mi (3.7 km), 1167 ft (356 m), the trail turns sharply southwest.

Proceed 0.8 mi (1.3 km) amid bluish-green mountain hemlock, pink-flowered alpine heather, and white granite while traversing beneath **Hidden Lake Peaks**— a serrated ridge. Flat rock slabs in a variety of shapes are ideal for sunning. The view from here is northwest to nearby Lookout Mtn and Monogram Peak, and to distant Mt. Baker.

The next stretch can hold snow as late as August. One snow gully is especially perilous; slip here and it could be your demise. That's why park rangers tend to say the lookout is inaccessible without an ice axe until mid-August.

After the switchback at 3.7 mi (6 km), you can see the lookout on the spire ahead, so you know where you're going even if you're walking atop snow. Just below that switchback, it's also possible to angle off trail (right / west), where the snow melts earlier and where you might feel more secure continuing the ascent. To do this, contour directly south, scrambling over dry rock and through heather, then angle back up left (southeast) to rejoin the trail at the 4-mi (6.4-km) point.

If the trail is buried, and both options—ascending the snowfields or routefinding—seem risky, you can turn back at 3.7 mi (6 km) feeling well rewarded for your effort. Keep in mind, snow here doesn't mean snow all the way to the lookout. The final 0.2 mi (0.3 km) melts out much earlier.

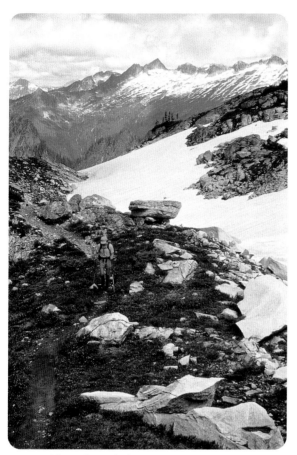

Near Hidden Lake Peaks lookout

At 4 mi (6.4 km) begin the last pitch: 700 ft (213 m) in 0.5 mi (0.8 km). At 4.2 mi (6.8 km) the trail turns left (east), passes a tiny tarn, and enters a narrow gully (possibly snow-filled, but not steep) directly beneath the lookout. At 4.3 mi (6.9 km) enter the **national park** and reach the notch between the lookout-crowned spire and the other Hidden Lake Peaks.

It's possible to scramble left (northeast) to the first of the peaks: 7088 ft (2160 m). For the lookout, turn right (southwest) and pick up the steep, narrow trail ascending the northeast side of the spire. Cairns indicate the route, switchbacking on packed dirt, boulders and slabs.

Reach the **summit** at 4.5 mi (7.2 km), 6900 ft (2103 m). The lookout cabin is anchored to a jumble of huge, blocky rocks.

Hidden Lake is visible 1167 ft (355 m) below you. The pinnacles of The Triad and the glacier-encrusted pyramid of 8868-foot (2703-m) Eldorado Peak are northeast. Forbidden Peak, Sahale Mtn, Boston Basin and Boston Glacier are east. Johannesburg Mtn is nearby southeast, above Cascade River Road. Mt. Formidable and Middle Cascade Glacier are southeast, looming above Cascade River's middle and south forks. Mt. Buckindy and Snowking Mtn are in the southern foreground, with Glacier Peak and Mt. Rainier behind them. Marblemount is northwest, in the Skagit River Valley. Sauk Mtn is farther west. The Easton Glacier and Railroad Grade are discernible on Mt. Baker, far north.

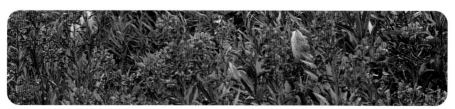

Fireweed

TRIP 30
BOSTON BASIN

LOCATION	North Cascades National Park
ROUND TRIP	8 mi (12.9 km)
ELEVATION GAIN	3000 ft (914 m)
KEY ELEVATIONS	trailhead 3200 ft (975 m), highpoint 6200 ft (1890 m)
HIKING TIME	6 to 7 hours
DIFFICULTY	challenging
MAPS	*Green Trails* Marblemount 47 (shows Cascade River road)
	Diablo Dam 48 (to identify peaks), Cascade Pass 80

OPINION

Water cascading over rocks all around you. Ice cascading down summits in every direction. A more Cascadian setting you will not find than this: the pinnacle-and-glacier amphitheater of Boston Basin.

Once in the alpine zone, slabs and moraines invite you to wander. Strike off in any direction, clambering over burnt-chili and fried-orange boulders that look like they tumbled out of the forge only moments ago. You can spend a full day exploring this new world, or enjoy a half day rock romping.

But before following the pull of the stone and ice above, turn your attention to the wonder of water. It's everywhere in Boston Basin. Try giving in, for just a moment, to water's gentle but persistent will. Lie down between creeklets. Close your eyes. Listen to the dribbling, gurgling, swishing liquid all around you—coursing over rock, through rock, under rock. It's cheerful music, delicate, almost fragile, yet it's one of the implacable forces that shaped these mountains.

The hike to Boston Basin begins on an old road, devolves into a vertical, rugged, slippery, climbers' route, then recovers a modicum of sanity as it rises steeply through big timber. It's easy to follow; it's just not easy to walk.

Give the snow plenty of time to melt before venturing here. On a year of normal snowfall, wait at least until late July. The less snow, the higher you can roam. And the less snow, the easier the unbridged stream crossings. Carry trekking poles for safer rockhopping and fording.

Pitching a tent in Boston Basin is an appealing idea, until you (1) consider the difficulty of hauling a full pack up that gnarly climbers' route, (2) remember how hard it is to find a level tentsite in such rocky terrain, and (3) realize that the basin's few sanctioned, established sites are constantly occupied by said climbers.

Better to start early, carry a daypack, go far, and stay only as long as the sun will allow.

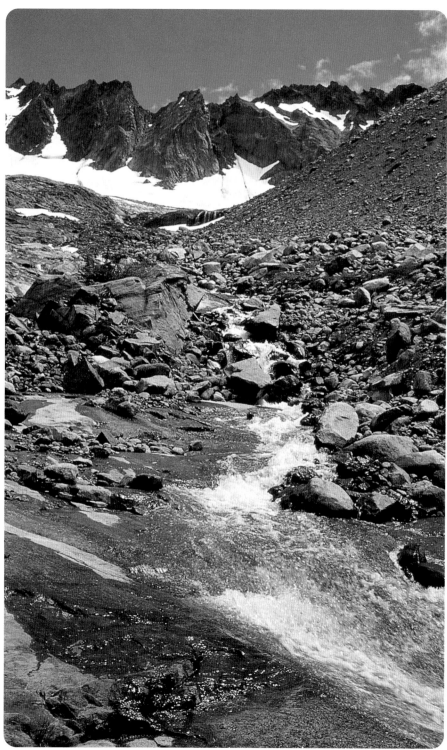

Boston Basin

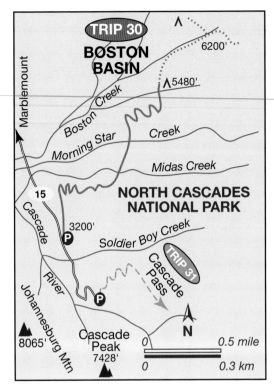

BY VEHICLE

At the east edge of Marble-mount, where Hwy 20 bends north, go straight (east) onto Cascade River Road and imme-diately cross the Skagit River. At 0.7 mi (1.1 km) pass the Rockport-Cascade Road on the right. Continue east on Cascade River Road 15. Pavement ends at 5.2 mi (8.4 km). At 8.3 mi (13.4 km) pass the entrance to Marble Creek campground. At 16.9 mi (27.2 km) curve sharply left, ignoring a right fork to the Cascade River trails. Enter the national park at 18.3 mi (29.5 km). Trailhead parking for Boston Basin is beside the road, on the left, at 22.8 mi (36.7 km), 3200 ft (975 m). If it's full, con-tinue to the spacious Cascade Pass trailhead parking lot at road's end: 23.5 mi (37.8 km), 3600 ft (1097 m).

ON FOOT

Initially follow an abandoned mining road generally north. Precisely where it departs the parking area might not be readily apparent. If necessary, part the brush that hides the entrance. What *is* apparent from the start is Johannesburg Mtn (southwest). It'll be visible and perhaps audible (ice fall) while you ascend.

Near 1 mi (1.6 km) glimpse your destination above (northeast) and Hidden Lake Peaks (west-northwest). The trail soon narrows to a bootbeaten path and steepens, climbing generally east. Expect it to be overgrown and per-haps cluttered with avalanche debris. To hoist yourself over rocks and roots, your feet will likely need help from your hands.

The grade does relent, however, and you'll soon be hiking again rather than scrambling. Your general direction of travel is north-northeast. Ahead: forest, avalanche swaths, and unbridged streams that require rockhopping (if you're lucky), fording (brrrrr), or the wisdom to forgo crossing if the runoff is torrential.

Beyond Midas and Morning Star creeks, enter the open lower reaches of **Boston Basin** at about 3 mi (4.8 km). You're now in wandering territory. Follow your bliss.

Vertical rock and ice is visible in all directions. Mt. Torment is north-northwest. West of it is Eldorado Creek pouring down the avalanche slope beneath Inspiration Glacier on the east side of Eldorado Peak. Forbidden Peak

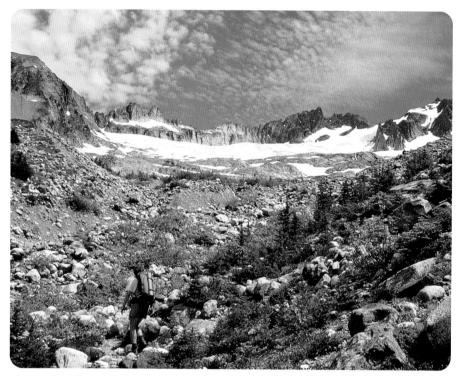

Approaching Boston Basin

is north. Boston Glacier is northeast. Boston Peak is east. Sahale Mtn is east-southeast. The Quien Sabe Glacier is between Boston Peak and Sahale Mtn.

Snow-level permitting, you can follow the climbers' path north then northeast. It crosses streams, ascends a moraine near Boston Creek, then forks at about 4 mi (6.4 km), 6200 ft (1890 m). Left quickly reaches tentsites among talus, between forks of Boston Creek. Right ascends toward the foot of Quien Sabe Glacier.

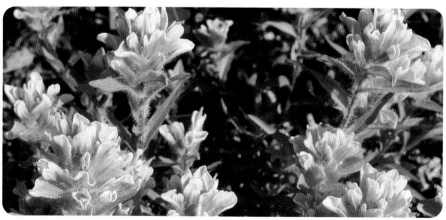

Less common, yellow paintbrush

TRIP 31
CASCADE PASS / SAHALE ARM

LOCATION	North Cascades National Park
ROUND TRIP	7.4 mi (11.9 km) to Cascade Pass
	12.4 mi (20 km) to Sahale camp
ELEVATION GAIN	1800 ft (549 m) to Cascade Pass
	5000 ft (1524 m) to Sahale camp
KEY ELEVATIONS	trailhead 3600 ft (1097 m), pass 5400 ft (1646 m)
	Sahale camp 6800 ft (2073 m)
HIKING TIME	3 to 6 hours
DIFFICULTY	moderate to challenging
MAP	*Green Trails* Cascade Pass 80

Here's the revival tent of North Cascades hikes. Want to convert athletic friends into hiking buddies? The trail to Cascade Pass is so short yet so scenic that its come-to-Jesus power is irresistible.

The sermonic views begin on the approach road, which is even more impressive than Hwy 20 through the national park. And towering above the trailhead are the cliffs and couloirs of 8065-ft (2458-m) Johannesburg Mtn—a sight as sublime as the culminating vistas on many other hikes.

Gently graded switchbacks make the initial climb—1400 ft (427 m) in 2.5 mi (4 km)—easier than it sounds. After that, a traversing ascent allows you to gaze at Johannesburg Mtn while you stride.

This trip's only drawback is its fame. Hundreds of boots pound the trail each summer weekend. Having to repeatedly chirp "hello" is a nuisance. On our way up one afternoon, we passed more than 50 people coming down.

By starting before 8 a.m. you can avoid most of the crowd and have time to wander up Sahale Arm. If you're going only as far the pass, start after 3 p.m. That way you'll have it mostly to yourself. And by descending around 6 or 7 p.m., you'll avoid the obligatory pleasantries.

To shake the crowd altogether, choose another hike, perhaps Boston Basin. Or just don't plop at the pass. Few people continue to the Doubtful Lake overlook. Fewer still attempt the arduous route to Sahale Glacier.

Beyond the pass, on the finger of Sahale Arm, you'll enter flowery meadows above Doubtful Lake—so named, we presume, because the bone-jarring descent to its lovely shores is a dubious enterprise. The view includes Eldorado Peak's Inspiration Glacier to the west.

Inspired? Press on. Leave the grassy slopes and continue ascending a steep, rocky moraine. The way gets sketchy, but the panorama keeps improving. Range upon range of spiky mountains to the south, including distant Glacier Peak, gradually reveal themselves.

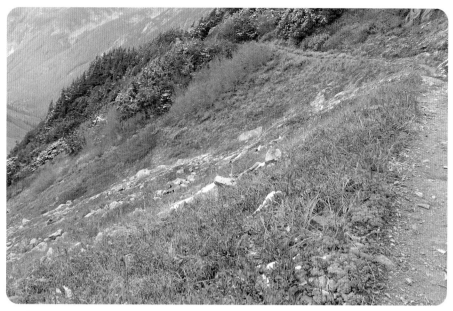

Trail to Cascade Pass, mid-September

You can walk, albeit knees to chest, all the way to Sahale Glacier. It's a challenging dayhike destination but poses no danger to hardy folk with a little scrambling experience. Further exploration onto the ice is for properly equipped climbers only.

FACT

BY VEHICLE

At the east edge of Marblemount, where Hwy 20 bends north, go straight (east) onto Cascade River Road and immediately cross the Skagit River. At 0.7 mi (1.1 km) pass the Rockport-Cascade Road on the right. Continue east on Cascade River Road 15. Pavement ends at 5.2 mi (8.4 km). At 8.3 mi (13.4 km) pass the entrance to Marble Creek campground. At 16.9 mi (27.2 km) curve sharply left, ignoring a right fork to the Cascade River trails. Enter the national park at 18.3 mi (29.5 km). At 23.5 mi (37.8 km) reach the spacious Cascade Pass trailhead parking lot at road's end, 3600 ft (1097 m).

ON FOOT

The trail to Cascade Pass is broad and well-maintained. A switchbacking ascent leads generally east-northeast through mature forest. Just over an hour up, at 2.5 mi (4 km), 5165 ft (1575 m), you're nearly out of the trees. Begin a long, gradual traverse south-southeast across alpine slopes. Reach **Cascade Pass** at 3.7 mi (6 km), 5400 ft (1646 m).

To see Doubtful Lake and explore Sahale Arm, don't continue on the main trail east-southeast into Pelton Basin. Follow the narrow trail starting just below the east side of Cascade Pass. Begin a switchbacking ascent generally north-northeast, up the ridge.

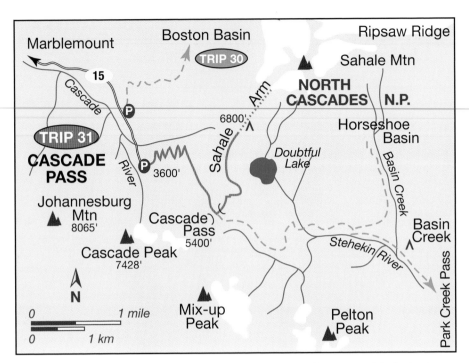

At 4.5 mi (7.2 km), 6100 ft (1859 m) you're on the crest of **Sahale Arm**. A spur descends about 800 ft (244 m) to Doubtful Lake. Your trail follows the meadowy ridgecrest—north, curving north-northeast toward Sahale Mtn. Where the greenery ends, follow the climbers' path ascending at a 45° angle atop the rocky moraine.

Reach campsites beneath Sahale Glacier at 6.2 mi (10 km), 6800 ft (2073 m). A national park backcountry camping permit is necessary to spend the night here.

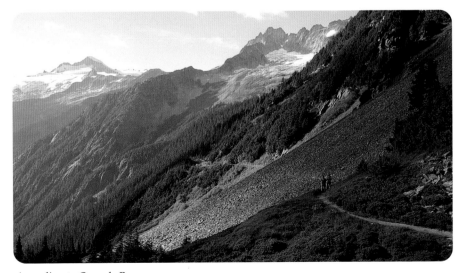

Ascending to Cascade Pass

TIFFANY MOUNTAIN

LOCATION	Okanogan National Forest
ROUND TRIP	6 mi (9.7 km)
ELEVATION GAIN	1742 ft (531 m)
KEY ELEVATIONS	trailhead 6500 ft (1981 m), summit 8242 ft (2512 m)
HIKING TIME	3 to 4 hours
DIFFICULTY	easy
MAP	*Green Trails* Tiffany Mtn 53

OPINION

On the northeast edge of the North Cascades stands a bare, rocky summit. It's so dry here, sunshine is almost a certainty in summer. There are no rivalling peaks in the neighborhood, so the vast views from the top are uneclipsed. The nearest highway is distant, so except for the buzz of an occasional insect or the swish of a breeze, soothing silence prevails. And because Tiffany Mtn is far from any sizeable town, you might happen upon the hiker's Holy Grail: solitude.

This shorn mountain is an anomaly among the shaggy, craggy alps dominating the range. The others are far more dramatic, but Tiffany is a different breed: softer, rounder, more welcoming.

Here, hiking feels like walking instead of climbing. And stopping to appreciate a blossom—of which there are many—is a prerogative instead of an excuse to catch your breath.

Though the summit is a respectable 8242 ft (2512 m) high and was even the site of a fire lookout from 1931 to 1953, you can assault it with your hands in your pockets. It's really a tilted, alpine meadow, studded with lichen-splotched granite boulders.

Precisely which blossoms might you admire here? Blue lupine, pastel-pink plumed avens, creamy-lime valerian, and yellow succulent stonecrop, to name a few.

What else might you see? The main range west. The Pasayten Wilderness north. The fertile farms of the Okanogan east. Tiffany Lake north-northwest.

You'll also see why you shouldn't hike anywhere else in the vicinity: surmounting treeline would require too long a tramp in forest.

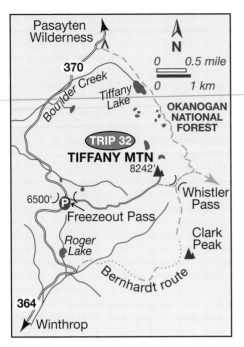

BY VEHICLE

Drive Hwy 20 to Winthrop. From the center of town, follow signs for Pearrygin Lake State Park. Proceed north on the East Chewuch River Road. Pass the state-park turnoff at 1.6 mi (2.6 km). At 6.6 mi (10.6 km), just before the road crosses the river, bear right onto Road 37 and continue north. At 7.9 mi (12.7 km), where Road 5010 forks left, stay right, heading northeast on Road 37. At 14 mi (22.5 km) stay right toward Roger Lake on Road 37. Pavement ends after the North Fork Boulder Creek bridge.

At a junction in 19.6 mi (31.5 km) go left (northeast) onto Road 39 toward Tiffany Spring. Pass the Bernhardt Mine trail at 21.1 mi (34 km) and the Roger Lake pullout just after. At 22.8 mi (36.7 km), 6500 ft (1981 m) arrive at Freezeout Pass and Freezeout trail 345 to Tiffany Mtn. Drive over the cattleguard and park along the right side of the road.

ON FOOT

Begin a moderate ascent east then southeast on Freezeout Ridge. The first 1.5 mi (2.4 km) are through open forest brightened by lupine. Trees soon give way to rocky meadowland scattered with granite boulders.

At 2 mi (3.2 km), the trail is braided. Stay on the main path. Don't angle left off-trail thinking that's a quicker way to the summit, which is now visible. The trail is more efficient. Generally, stay closer to the right (south) side of the ridge until the trail, sometimes a shallow trench, clearly cuts left, ascending north among rocks and tussock.

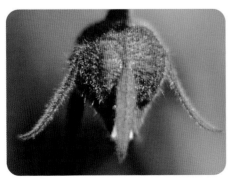

At 2.5 mi (4 km) you might notice a faint trail beginning to contour right (northeast). Ignore it. It goes to Whistler Pass. Bear left (north) now on a rough but obvious trail to reach the former fire-lookout site atop **Tiffany Mtn** at 3 mi (4.8 km), 8242 ft (2512 m).

Countless peaks are visible on the horizon. West and a bit south is Kangaroo Ridge near Washington Pass, as well as Silver Star and Gardner mountains. West are Goat Peak,

Plumed aven

Mt. Ballard, and Robinson Mtn. Southwest are the peaks rising above Twisp River valley. North are the mountains along the Boundary Trail, west of Horseshoe Basin. East is Okanogan farmland.

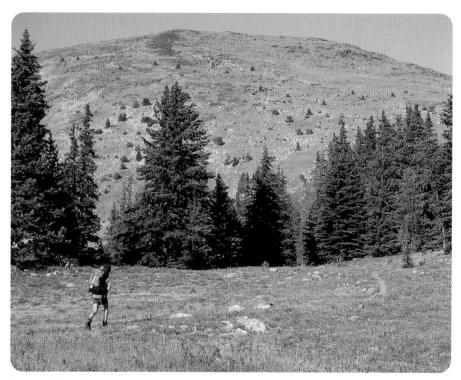

Tiffany Mountain

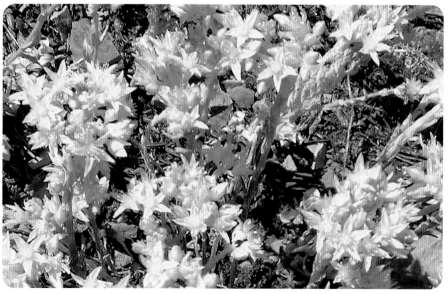

Stonecrop

TRIP 33

TWISP PASS / STILLETO LAKE

LOCATION   Okanogan National Forest / Lake Chelan-Sawtooth
Wilderness / North Cascades National Park
ROUND TRIP   8.4 mi (13.5 km) to Twisp Pass
10.4 mi (16.7 km) to Stilleto Lake
ELEVATION GAIN   2400 ft (732 m) to Twisp Pass, 3100 ft (945 m) to Stilleto Lake
KEY ELEVATIONS   trailhead 3700 ft (1128 m), Twisp Pass 6100 ft (1859 m)
Stilleto Lake 6800 ft (2073 m)
HIKING TIME   4 to 5 hours for Twisp Pass, 5 to 6 hours for Stilleto Lake
DIFFICULTY   easy to Twisp Pass, moderate to Stilleto Lake
MAP   *Green Trails* Stehekin 82

OPINION

Airy trails—atop ridges or across cliffs, with at least one side open to a deep expanse—are thrilling. En route to Twisp Pass you'll reach a wonderfully long, airy stretch within a couple miles. It affords a continuous view of swooping, pinnacled peaks.

From the pass, an exhilarating high route continues, allowing you to roam alplands to Stilleto Lake, continue to a former fire-lookout site on the shoulder of Stilleto Peak, and perhaps complete a circuit via Copper Pass.

Meadows, creeklets, rock gardens, larches, and glimpses of a dozen mammoth mountains make the extended journey beyond Twisp Pass the most rewarding in the eastern reaches of the North Cascades. Big bonus: it's often dry and sunny here while it's sodden and grey farther west.

Hiking to Twisp Pass and back requires only about a half a day. An out-and-back hike past Stilleto Lake to the old Stilleto lookout is a full day's adventure. Only ambitious hikers—strong and fast, nimble on trackless terrain—should attempt to see the lake, tag the lookout, and return via Copper Pass before sunset.

Perusing a map, you might zero-in on Dagger Lake as your destination. But gazing down on it from just above Twisp Pass, you'll realize it's better to stay high than plummet to the lake's forested shores. Stilleto Lake is a much more gratifying goal.

Carry one full water bottle more than you imagine you'll need. It's a hot day? Carry two more than you think you'll need. If you don't drop to Dagger Lake, you can count on refilling only twice: at the 1.7-mi (2.7-km) trail junction, and at Stilleto Lake.

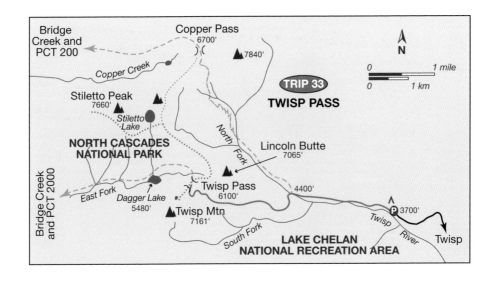

Bridge
Creek and
PCT 200

Copper Pass
6700'

▲▲7840'

Copper Creek

Stiletto Peak
7660' ▲▲

·Stiletto·
·Lake·

North Fork

TRIP 33
TWISP PASS

0   1 mile
0   1 km

N

NORTH CASCADES
NATIONAL PARK

Lincoln Butte
7065'

▲

Bridge Creek
and PCT 2000

East Fork

Dagger Lake
5480'

Twisp Pass
6100'

4400'

▲Twisp Mtn
7161'

South Fork

LAKE CHELAN
NATIONAL RECREATION AREA

Twisp River

Twisp

3700'

FACT

BY VEHICLE

Drive Hwy 20—south from Winthrop, or east from Okanogan—to Twisp. Turn west onto the paved Twisp River Road, signed for Twisp River Rec Area. At 11 mi (17.7 km) reach a junction. Proceed straight (northwest) on Twisp River Road. At 14.6 mi (23.5 km) the road forks. Continue straight. Pass the official North Creek / Twisp Pass trailhead on the right at 25 mi (40.2 km).

Reach Road's End campground at 25.6 mi (41.2 km), 3700 ft (1128 m). By starting here, rather than at the official trailhead, you can shorten your round-trip hiking distance by 0.8 mi (1.3 km). If you're not camping, don't park in a campsite.

ON FOOT

Look behind the outhouses for a bootbeaten path vaulting up the hillside. Quickly intersect the trail, turn left, and hike generally west-northwest.

Following the Twisp River upstream, the trail is high above the north bank. It ascends through forest and dense brush with a sprinkling of wildflowers. Though horses are allowed, the narrow trail is infrequently ridden and the surface is rocky, so dust and mud are not a problem.

After gaining 700 ft (213 m) in 1.7 mi (2.7 km), reach a junction at 4400 ft (1341 m). Stay left for Twisp Pass. Right leads northwest 4 mi (6.4 km) to Copper Pass; you'll return that way if you hike a cross-country circuit linking Twisp and Copper. Refill water bottles here, because water is scarce beyond.

Turning left, immediately cross a footlog spanning the **North Fork Twisp River**—a mere creek. The trail then darts upward, gaining 200 ft (61 m) in 0.1 mi (0.2 km), before abruptly turning left (south) and contouring around the east ridge of Lincoln Butte.

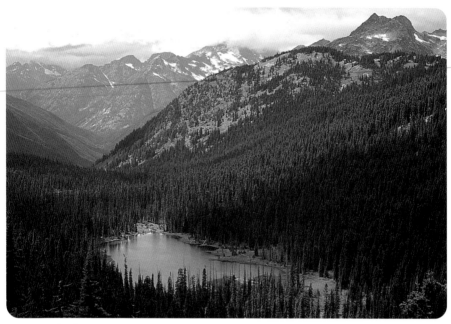

Dagger Lake, from Twisp Pass

Heading generally west, at 2.1 mi (3.4 km) enjoy views south, across the South Fork Twisp River valley to the peaks beyond. Smooth rock slabs suggest it's time for a scenic rest break. Hock Mtn, with its serrated summit ridge and lush avalanche slopes, is soon visible at the head of the valley.

After 2.5 mi (4 km) the trail curves northwest, ascending steadily. Open, rocky slopes grant views. Though blasted out of a cliffside, the airy trail affords secure, comfortable passage. Crest 6100-ft (1859-m) **Twisp Pass** at 4.2 mi (6.8 km), on the North Cascades National Park boundary. Dagger Lake is visible ahead (west-northwest) 620 ft (189 m) below, at 5480 ft (1670 m). Forested Bridge Creek valley is farther west.

The trail drops to Dagger Lake then continues west, down-valley to Bridge Creek, where it intersects the Pacific Crest Trail. After attaining an aerial view of Dagger, however, why descend into forest?

From the pass, it's possible to follow the ridgecrest less than 0.5 mi (0.8 km) southwest to a tiny lake near the base of Twisp Mtn. You might also ascend a bootbeaten route into the rocky meadows northeast of the pass for views of Goode Mtn (west) and Mt. Logan (northwest).

Given time, energy and desire, keep following the route northwest through alpine parkland—grassy benches peppered with boulders, splashed with wildflowers—to **Stiletto Lake** at 5.2 mi (8.4 km), 6800 ft (2073 m), in a cirque beneath Stiletto Peak.

It's even possible to continue out Stiletto's west buttress and ascend to where a fire lookout once stood at 7220 ft (2200 m), less than a mile from the lake. From there you can look north-northeast to Liberty Bell and the Early Winters Spires, north to Tower Mtn, and northwest to Black Peak and Mt. Arriva.

Copper Pass is north-northeast of Stiletto Lake, less than a mile distant. It's a cross-country ramble that simply requires you to maintain your elevation as much as possible while hiking in that general direction. It's not difficult for experienced navigators, but start early, carry a topo map and compass, and refill water bottles at the lake.

Upon intersecting the trail at 6700-ft (2042-m) **Copper Pass**, turn right. Follow it southeast 4 mi (6.4 km) down the North Fork to the junction with the Twisp Pass trail, where you're again on familiar ground. Left here leads 1.7 mi (2.7 km) east-southeast to the trailhead.

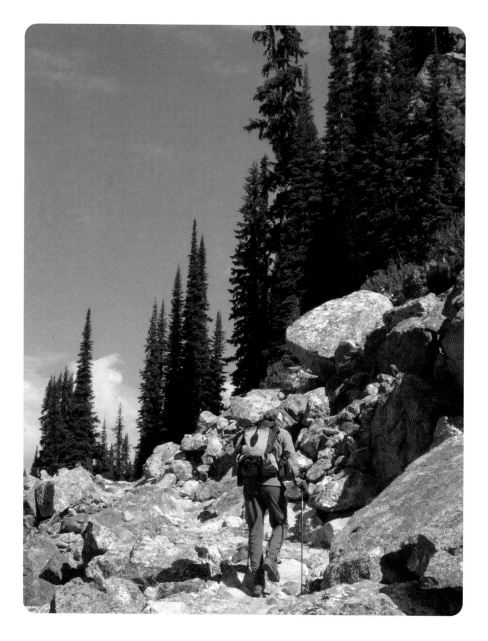

TRIP 34
GREEN MOUNTAIN

LOCATION	Mt. Baker-Snoqualmie National Forest
	Glacier Peak Wilderness
ROUND TRIP	8 mi (12.9 km)
ELEVATION GAIN	3000 ft (914 m)
KEY ELEVATIONS	trailhead 3500 ft (1067 m), Green Mtn 6500 ft (1981 m)
HIKING TIME	4 to 5 hours
DIFFICULTY	moderate
MAP	*Green Trails* Cascade Pass 80

The restored 1933 fire lookout cabin crowning Green Mtn is a superb aerie. You can peer into deep, forested valleys brooding below, and gaze across at brazen peaks challenging the heavens.

Gentle switchbacks and ever-expanding scenery ease your passage to the summit. Nearby north is an unnamed Tahitian-green pyramidal mountain. Farther north is Mt. Buckindy. To the east, you can trace the courses of Downey and Bachelor creeks below you, and above see an ambitious mountaineering route: the Ptarmigan Traverse from glacier-capped Dome Peak, north to Mt. Formidable. Dominating the southeast horizon is Glacier Peak.

The first couple miles of the Green Mtn trail are usually snow-free in May. That's far enough to appreciate the annual spring flush of glacier lilies and high enough to spy Dome and Glacier peaks. But snow in the basin beneath the summit usually stops hikers until July.

From mid-July to early August, you can stalk tigers here. The spotted, orange, docile ones: tiger lilies. These exotic-looking blossoms speckle the greenery all the way up the south-facing slope. Other species thrive here as well, including Sitka

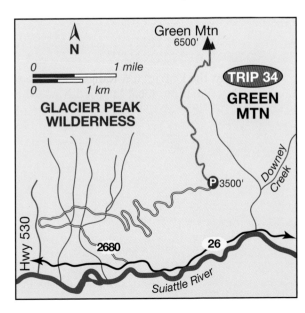

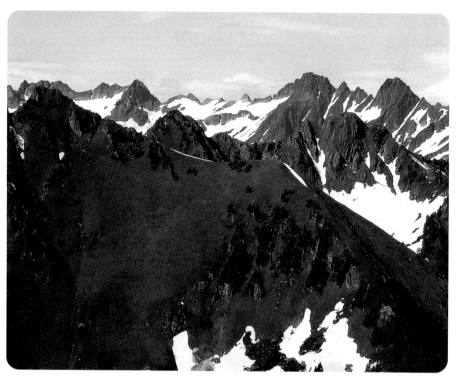

Glacier Peak Wilderness, from Green Mountain

valerian, purple penstemon, and columbine. This resplendent display rivals any in the North Cascades.

FACT

BY VEHICLE

Drive Hwy 530 south 11.3 mi (18.2 km) from Rockport, or north 7.2 mi (11.6 km) from the Darrington Ranger Station. Turn east onto Suiattle River Road 26. Proceed 19 mi (30.6 km) southeast, then turn left onto Green Mtn Road 2680. Just before it ends, park at 24.8 mi (39.9 km), 3500 ft (1067 m), where the signed trail departs left. From the road you can survey the Suiattle River valley. Downey Mtn, directly east, splits Sulphur and Downey creeks.

ON FOOT

A switchbacking ascent generally north through mossy forest emerges at 1 mi (1.6 km) among lime-green corn lilies, wildflowers, tall grass, then blueberry bushes. Already you can see White Chuck Mtn (southwest), Sloan Peak (south), and Glacier Peak (southeast).

At 2 mi (3.2 km), 5200 ft (1585 m), Dome Peak is visible east. Farther southeast are Plummer and Fortress mountains, above Suiattle Pass. The trail then leaves this south-facing slope, rounds the end of a ridge, then resumes north, dropping 150 ft (46 m) to shallow **tarns** in fragile meadows.

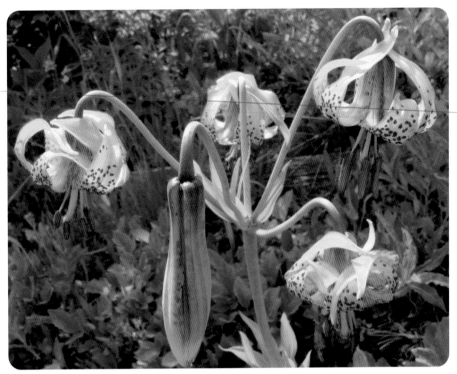

Tiger lilies abound on Green Mountain.

Here on the shady north side of the ridge, snow lingers many weeks longer than on the south slope. Though the braided, eroded trail is slippery when wet, try not to initiate yet another path.

Above the tarns, enter a **basin**—probably snow covered until mid-July—where you can see the trail slicing toward the summit. Carry on—northeast then north—and at 4 mi (6.4 km), 6500 ft (1981 m), you'll be standing atop **Green Mtn**.

Condemned in 1995, the Green Mtn fire lookout cabin was restored in 1999 with a grant from the White House Millennium Council's *Saving America's Treasures* program. It was pushed off its foundation in 2001, however, by a huge snow cornice.

In pieces, it was airlifted to Darrington where it was rebuilt. By late 2007 it should again be atop the mountain and open to the public, but check with the Darrington Ranger Station to be sure.

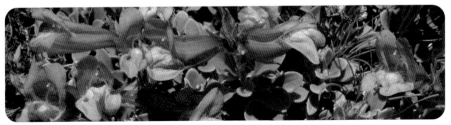

Penstemon

LAKE TWENTYTWO

LOCATION	Lake 22 Research Natural Area
ROUND TRIP	5.4 mi (8.7 km)
ELEVATION GAIN	1313 ft (400 m)
KEY ELEVATIONS	trailhead 1100 ft (335 m), lake 2413 ft (735 m)
HIKING TIME	2 to 3 hours
DIFFICULTY	easy
MAPS	*Green Trails* Granite Falls 109, Silverton 110

OPINION

Lake 22 Research Natural Area is a 980-acre (397-hectare) haven of virgin forest in a region of profligate logging. It was protected in 1947 for an absurd reason: to see if a preserved forest would, over time, flourish more than a similar forest "under intensive management," in other words, a forest that's been plundered. We all know the answer, and the pure, raw beauty you'll experience on this hike elaborates eloquently. So chalk this up as one time we've benefitted from the government's lack of common sense.

The trail was smartly engineered and is well maintained. Thanks to the gravel surface, even during a downpour you won't be tromping in mud or sloshing through water. You'll be striding among resplendent ancient cedars and hemlocks, often beside a gorgeous creek. Several waterfalls add to the enchantment. You'll enjoy the revitalizing walk as much as the beautiful destination: an impressive glacial cirque, with ribbon waterfalls gracing the luxuriant green cliffs that rise from the lakeshore straight up the north flank of Mt. Pilchuck.

Because it's at only 2413 ft (735 m), Lake Twentytwo is accessible most of the year. It makes an excellent rainy-day hike, because you'll still be able to appreciate the scenery. Cloud and mist actually enhance it, creating a mysterious, primeval atmosphere. In early spring, you'll likely witness avalanches crashing into the lake. You'll be safe on the north shore, across from the cliffs. In early October, the nearly half-mile stretch of trail through maple trees is a collage of blazing fall colors. So shoulder season is preferable to mid-summer, when this easy trail attracts droves of walkers.

FACT

BY VEHICLE

From the Verlot Public Service Center, drive the Mountain Loop Hwy east 2.1 mi (3.4 km). Turn right (south) into the spacious, circular, trailhead parking lot at 1100 ft (335 m).

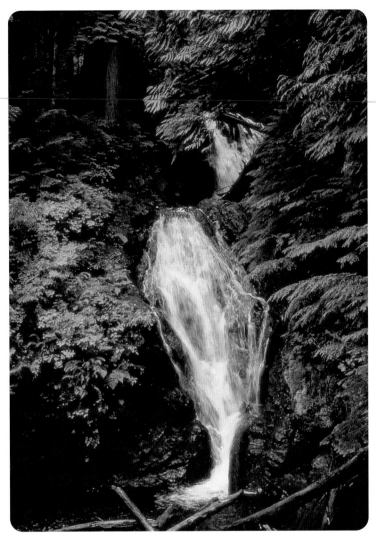

Cascade en route to Lake Twentytwo

ON FOOT

Immediately cross the bridge spanning **Hempel Creek** and head west into an ancient hemlock-and-cedar forest. Soon begin a switchbacking ascent. At 0.75 mi (1.2 km) cross the bridge spanning **22 Creek**. At a moderate grade, the trail switchbacks generally southwest through ancient forest, past several waterfalls.

The third and biggest falls is at 1.3 mi (2.1 km), just off the trail. When you hear a roar, look left through the trees and you'll see it. To get closer, find the rocky spur veering off a tight switchback where the trail doubles back from east to west. This is 0.2 mi (0.3 km) before the trail crosses a rockslide among maples.

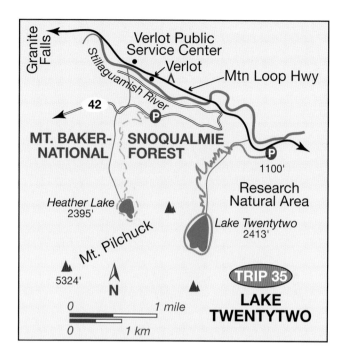

If you miss the third falls going up, you'll probably catch it on the way down. From the rockslide, the heavily clearcut South Fork Stillaguamish River valley is visible north. The final approach to your destination is southward.

At 2.7 mi (4.3 km), 2413 ft (735 m) reach the north shore of **Lake Twentytwo**. A trail with sections of helpful boardwalk circles the lake.

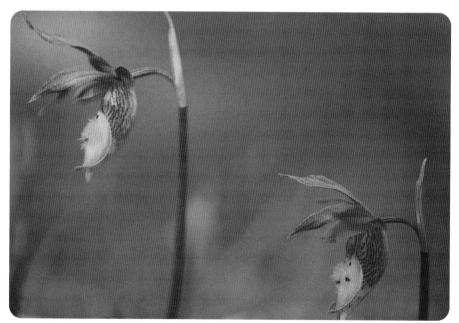

In spring, look for Calypso orchids (also called fairyslipper*) in forests.*

TRIP 36

MT. DICKERMAN

LOCATION	Mt. Baker-Snoqualmie National Forest
ROUND TRIP	8.6 mi (13.8 km)
ELEVATION GAIN	3923 ft (1196 m)
KEY ELEVATIONS	trailhead 1800 ft (549 m), Mt. Dickerman 5723 ft (1744 m)
HIKING TIME	4½ to 5½ hours
DIFFICULTY	moderate
MAP	*Green Trails* Sloan Peak 111

OPINION

Gazing straight up at Mt. Dickerman from the trailhead is enough to blow out your aorta. It looks like a brutally steep hike, for masochists only. So just keep your head down and go. The trail is well engineered, the switchbacks gentle. The unmolested, ancient forest is inspiring. After just 2.5 mi (4 km) the views are extensive. On top, the 360° panorama is exhilarating.

On a clear day, the summit offers a visual feast. (The profuse blueberries just below are a tasty hors d'oeuvre, or perhaps dessert.) You can see all the peaks rising above the Mountain Loop Hwy, towering above the South Fork Stillaguamish and Sauk river valleys, plus many more.

Strong hikers can gallop up Dickerman in a little over two hours. But regardless of pace, hikers enjoy this surprisingly sensible, well-maintained trail. Allow at least an hour on top to gorge on the scenery. The time will race, especially if you enjoy identifying peaks.

Solitude is unlikely. Even on a weekday during a very rainy October, eight people paid homage to the North Cascades atop Dickerman. Mid-September to mid-October, when the blueberries are ripe and the bushes are resplendent

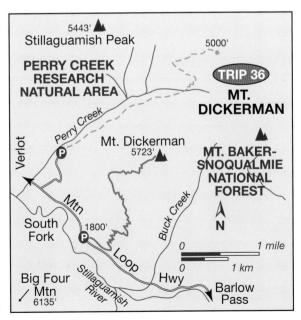

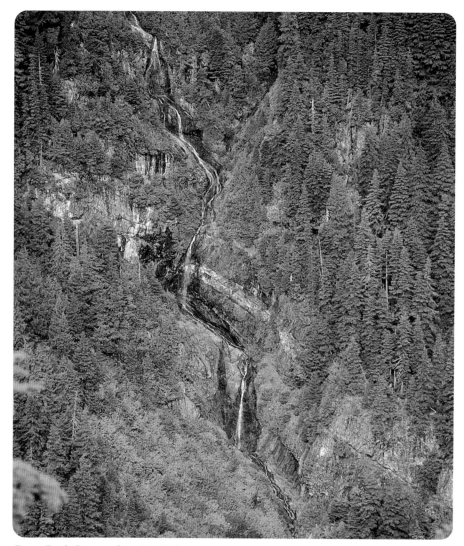

Perry Creek Canyon, from Mt. Dickerman ascent

red, is the ideal time to come. If you're lucky, you'll be here after a brief autumn snowfall has dusted the peaks, accentuating the crags.

FACT

BY VEHICLE

Drive the Mountain Loop Hwy southeast 16.7 mi (26.9 km) from the Verlot Public Service Center, or northwest 3 mi (4.8 km) from Barlow Pass. The small trailhead parking lot is on the northeast side of the highway, at 1800 ft (549 m).

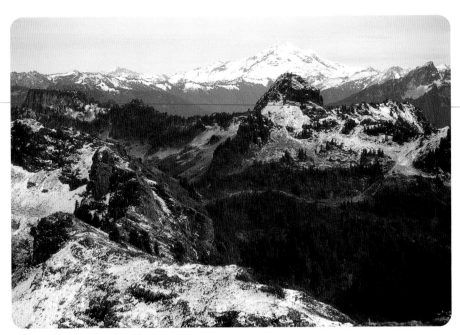

Glacier Peak, from Mt. Dickerman

ON FOOT

A switchbacking ascent leads generally north-northeast among cedars and subalpine firs. The taxing grade soon relents slightly. The roar of unseen water is audible the first couple miles.

At 2.6 mi (4.2 km) Big Four Mtn is visible southwest across the valley. Near 3 mi (4.8 km) pass beneath broken cliffs and arrive at a small waterfall and pool. After a level respite, the trail turns sharply east. Watch for a short left spur leading west to an overlook above Perry Creek drainage.

The last mile is steep, but views expand with every step. The final ascent is generally northeast. Reach the 5723-ft (1744-m) summit of **Mt. Dickerman** at 4.3 mi (6.9 km).

Ah, the view. To the northwest are Three Fingers and Whitehorse Mtn, with Mts. Baker and Shuksan in the background. Mt. Forgotten is immediately north. White Chuck and Pugh mountains are just beyond. To the northeast, Lost Creek Ridge angles toward Glacier Peak. To the east are Sloan Peak and the Monte Cristo group. Southeast are the snow-capped peaks of Alpine Lakes Wilderness. Nearby to the south are, from left to right, Del Campo, Morning Star, and Sperry. Big Four is also close, southwest. Mt. Rainier is way south. To the southwest are Mt. Pilchuck, Puget Sound, and the Olympic Range rising abruptly from the sea.

TRIP 37

GOAT LAKE

SHOULDER SEASON

LOCATION	Mt. Baker-Snoqualmie National Forest
	Henry M. Jackson Wilderness
ROUND TRIP	10.4 mi (16.7 km)
ELEVATION GAIN	1261 ft (384 m)
KEY ELEVATIONS	trailhead 1900 ft (579 m), lake 3161 ft (963 m)
HIKING TIME	4 to 5 hours
DIFFICULTY	easy
MAP	*Green Trails* Sloan Peak 111

OPINION

Mountain magnificence attainable in May? Yes. Low elevation and southern exposure enable you to hike beneath saw-toothed, snow-capped peaks into the tremendous Goat Lake cirque, where you can safely watch avalanches crash down Foggy Peak. It's an exhilarating change from the viewless, deep-forest walks that are the usual early-season fare.

Goat Lake cirque is sufficiently beautiful to justify a summer visit. Heat and crowds, however, will detract from the experience. And of course, by then, more rewarding challenges are available at higher elevations. Better to come early and feel the thrill of stealing into forbidden territory. If you do come in summer, carry sufficient water, because all the convenient trail-side sources (fed by snowmelt) will have vanished.

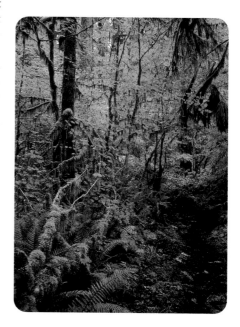

En route you'll pass goliath cedars that, to an open mind and appreciative eye, can be as emotionally moving as great mountains. The cedars, after all, are alive. They breathe. You encounter them intimately. By comparison, stone monoliths can seem cold, hard, distant, detached.

The trail to Goat Lake is usually hikeable by May 1, even in years of average snowfall. But until it's been brushed, expect to negotiate copious deadfall, or perhaps "livingfall." Six times we were forced to clamber over and under toppled trees burgeoning with spring growth. The steep slopes above the trail tend to slump during torrential rains, humiliating the poor trees in the process.

The trail reaches Goat Lake where its outlet stream, Elliott Creek, begins life as a waterfall. Continue along the forested northeast shore to find several private, rocky, pocket beaches, just big enough for two or three friends to lunch and snooze beside the lapping water. On a sunny spring day, it's heavenly here. And the Goat Lake campsites are near the outlet, within earshot of the soothing rumble of the falls.

Be aware that two paths depart the Goat Lake trailhead. The one described here is more popular. Though a former logging road and a mile longer, it's higher, drier, less subject to deadfall and erosion, thus easier to walk. It also grants views of the surrounding topography. The more direct alternative stays lower, following Elliot Creek upstream (southeast). The paths merge 1.6 mi (2.6 km) shy of the lake. Even the one described here can present obstacles after a hard winter, so expect more difficulties along Elliot Creek.

FACT

BY VEHICLE

From Darrington, drive the Mountain Loop Hwy southeast 19.8 mi (31.9 km) toward Barlow Pass. (Pavement ends at 9.5 mi / 15.3 km). Or, from the east side of Granite Falls, drive the Mountain Loop Hwy east 30.75 mi (49.5 km) to Barlow Pass, then continue northeast 3.5 mi (5.6 km). From either approach, turn east onto Elliot Creek Road 4080 and proceed 1 mi (1.6 km) to the road's end trailhead at 1900 ft (579 m).

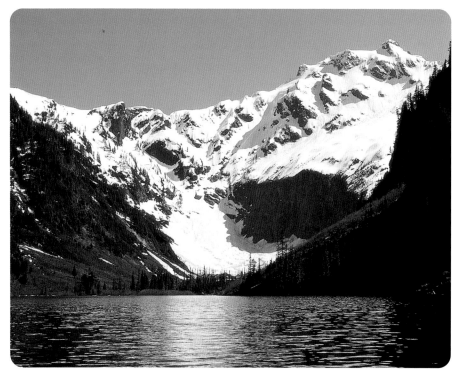

Goat Lake in May

A broad, smooth path—trail 647, actually a former logging road—heads generally southeast. Within 0.3 mi (0.5 km) it veers left and proceeds generally north. A long waterfall is visible on Twin Peaks, across Sauk River valley.

Mostly in alder, the road traverses above an old clearcut. At 1 mi (1.6 km) fork right, following the road south. It gradually curves southeast. Near 3.6 mi (5.8 km) it narrows to trail.

At 4.3 mi (6.9 km) enter the Henry M. Jackson Wilderness. You're now in a lush forest harboring many ancient cedars. It's cooler here than on the previous stretch among deciduous trees.

Continually showered with pine needles, the trail can blur into the forest floor. Stay alert to avoid straying off. Near the signed National Forest boundary, bear left on a gentle switchback, stepping over two boulders in the rocky channel. Right at this false junction plows into deadfall.

At 5 mi (8 km) reach roaring **Elliot Creek** spilling from **Goat Lake**. The lake is just beyond at 5.2 mi (8.4 km), 3161 ft (963 m). Treed campsites are uphill (left), where a hotel once stood. Camping is prohibited within 200 ft (61 m) of the lake.

The north ridge of 6810-ft (2076-m) Foggy Peak plunges to the lake's southwest shore, and 7186-ft (2190-m) Cadet Peak is visible above the south shore. A narrow, brushy path follows the northeast shore past tiny beaches to a waterfall and a cove halfway up the lake.

TRIP 38
GOTHIC BASIN

LOCATION	Mt. Baker-Snoqualmie National Forest
	Department of Natural Resources
ROUND TRIP	9.4 mi (15.1 km)
ELEVATION GAIN	2639 ft (804 m)
KEY ELEVATIONS	trailhead 2361 ft (720 m), basin 5000 ft (1524 m)
HIKING TIME	4½ to 6 hours
DIFFICULTY	moderate
MAPS	*Green Trails* Sloan Peak 111, Monte Cristo 143

OPINION

Gothic Basin is chaos set in stone. Come here to wander among patches of greenery dotted with ferns and flowers in a dramatically stark, rocky arena reminiscent of the Scottish Highlands.

Gothic is more interesting than nearby Glacier Basin. You can happily roam here for hours. Even the approach is enjoyable. After a stint in forest, you're on a long, high traverse, with open views, cooling breezes, plentiful water, and few flies.

The easy-to-follow trail is only moderately strenuous into the basin. From there, pick your way up to the surprisingly large Foggy Lake and continue

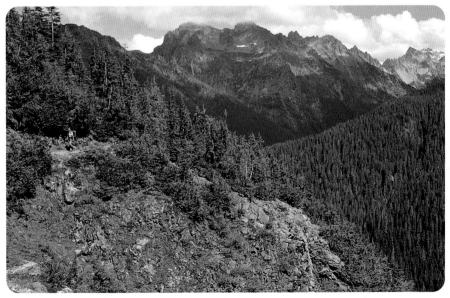

Monte Cristo peaks, from beneath Del Campo Peak

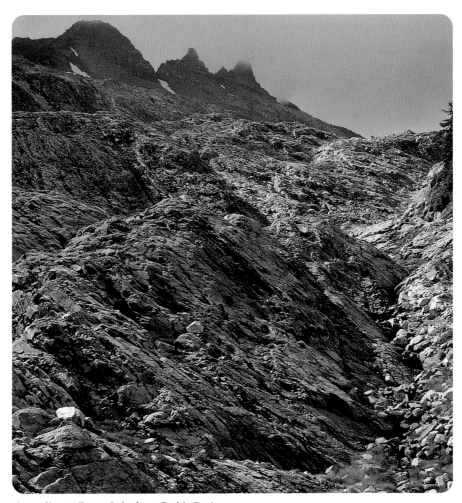

Ascending to Foggy Lake from Gothic Basin

beyond to Foggy Pass—easy to reach on a vigorous dayhike if you start reasonably early.

Approaching Foggy Lake's south shore, you'll see a boulder slope left (southwest). Go. The top affords a tremendous view of ragged pinnacles, the Sultan River drainage below, and mountains marching south to Stevens Pass.

FACT

BY VEHICLE

Drive the Mountain Loop Hwy—23.7 mi (38.1 km) southeast from Darrington, or 19.8 mi (31.9 km) east then southeast from the Verlot Public Service Center—to signed Barlow Pass. Park off the highway, or in the lot on the north side, at 236l ft (720 m).

ON FOOT

Follow the gated dirt road south toward Monte Cristo. At 1.2 mi (1.9 km), 2400 ft (732 m), just before the bridge spanning the **South Fork Sauk River**, turn right onto the signed Gothic Basin trail.

After a gentle stretch, ascend south through deep forest. At 2.75 mi (4.4 mi), the trail begins a steep traverse south-southwest on open slopes beneath Del Campo Peak. Soon cross a couple creeklets and pass a cool cascade. Silvertip Peak is visible southeast across Weden Creek. Farther east, above Glacier Basin, are Cadet, Monte Cristo, and Kyes peaks.

The ascent eases for 0.7 mi (1.1 km), but is again steep and rough at 3.6 mi (5.8 km). Heather and flowers brighten the way. Enter **Gothic Basin** at 4.7 mi (7.6 km), 5000 ft (1524 m). Immediately northwest is 6213-ft (1894-m) Gothic Peak.

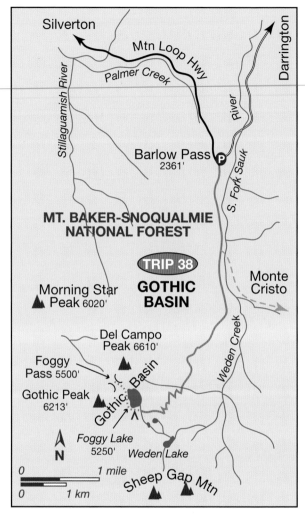

A fascinating variety of rock—bared and polished by the glacier that lived here long ago—enhances the beauty of this alpine basin. The predominate brown limestone has been weathered into strange shapes. You'll also see sandstone, conglomerate, granite, and iron-red mineralized zones.

Proceed north-northwest up either side of the creekbed to reach **Foggy Lake** at 5250 ft (1600 m). Round the west shore and resume ascending northwest on slabs and talus to arrive at 5500-ft (1676-m) **Foggy Pass**. Between Del Campo Peak (northeast) and Gothic Peak (southwest), the pass affords an impressive view of nearby Morning Star Peak (northwest).

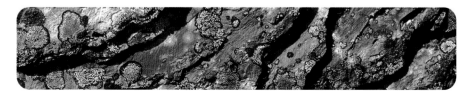

BLANCA LAKE

LOCATION	Mt. Baker-Snoqualmie National Forest
	Henry M. Jackson Wilderness
ROUND TRIP	8 mi (12.9 km) to Blanca Lake
ELEVATION GAIN	2700 ft (823 m) to ridge above Blanca Lake
	plus 628 ft (191 m) return from the lake
KEY ELEVATIONS	trailhead 1900 ft (579 m), highpoint 4600 ft (1402 m)
	lake 3972 ft (1211 m)
HIKING TIME	5 to 6 hours
DIFFICULTY	moderate
MAP	*Green Trails* Monte Cristo 143

OPINION

Blanca Lake's cloudy surface reflecting the surrounding shaggy cliffs is like an impressionist painting. With imaginative eyes you'll see the colors of an Italian piazza: chartreuse, siena, charcoal, salmon. But the setting—a dramatic cirque beneath towering Columbia Peak—takes no imagination to appreciate. The magnificence of it clubs you over the head.

Yet this isn't merely a trudge to a climactic viewpoint; it's a rich experience overall. The textures and hues of the forest and understory en route are as captivating as Blanca's deep bowl and awesome headwall.

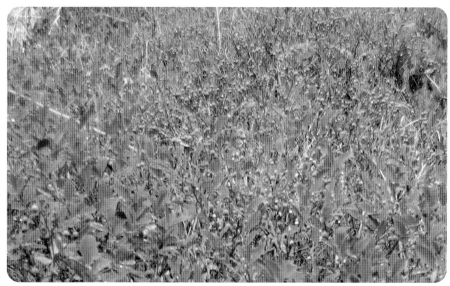

Profuse berries in early September along Blanca Lake trail

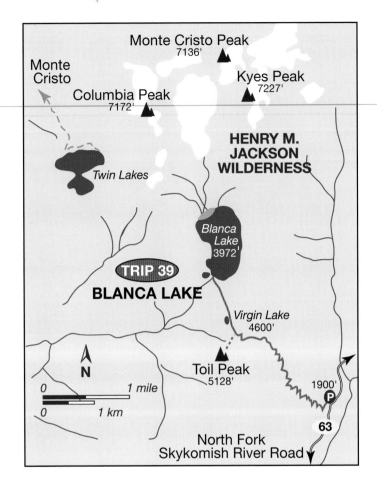

The thriving flora seems on the verge of taking over the trail completely. In September, you can feast along the way on a bumper crop of sweet, juicy berries. The ridge harbors curious pocket meadows. When fog is sifting through the canopy here, "Costa Rican cloud forest" springs to mind.

The steep trail switchbacks countless times. Anyone less than fit will feel the crack of the whip on this ascent. And other than a glimpse of Glacier Peak, there are no inspiring vistas until the Blanca Lake overlook. But the beauty of the immediate surroundings is carrot enough.

Even after heavy rain, the trail should be in good shape. That, plus the fact that your destination isn't a sky-high perch, make this a good choice during overcast weather.

After passing Virgin Lake (actually a pond), you'll see Columbia Glacier while descending toward milky teal Blanca Lake. It looks like one you'd have to fly into. (Be careful on the steep descent, or you just might.) The vast, seemingly bottomless chasm to your left is nearly as captivating as the lake and glacier.

Lots of people camp at Blanca, yet there's little room. *Crampground* is more like it. Rain or shine, expect to see tents jammed into the few sites near the log-strewn shore and among the boulders across the outlet stream. It's better to

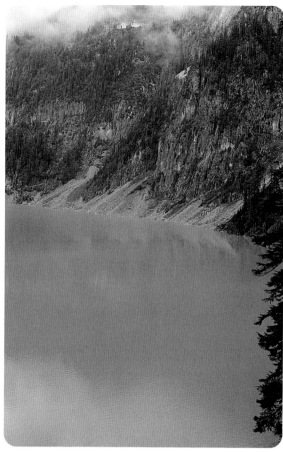

Blanca Lake

dayhike. You'll bank a little extra energy by not hauling a full pack. Spend it on some earnest scrambling around the west shore, in search of privacy, or on an aerial-view detour to Toil Peak.

BY VEHICLE

Drive Hwy 2 to Index. It's east of Monroe, northwest of Skykomish. Don't cross the bridge into the town. Follow paved North Fork Skykomish River Road 63 northeast 14.5 mi (23.3 km) to a junction. Bear left, staying on Road 63. Pavement ends. Reach the signed Blanca Lake trailhead parking area on the left at 16.7 mi (26.9 km), 1900 ft (579 m).

ON FOOT

The trail starts at the far end of the parking lot and immediately begins ascending steeply. The switchbacks lead generally northwest. The grade is aggressive: nearly 1000 ft/mi (305 m/1.6 km).

After angling north-northwest, then veering west, the trail crests a **ridge** and enters Henry M. Jackson Wilderness at 3 mi (4.8 km), 4600 ft (1402 m).

Shortly past tiny Virgin Lake, your destination is visible below (north). Beyond and above it is Columbia Glacier, between Columbia Peak (left) and Monte Cristo and Kyes peaks (right).

The trail then descends north-northwest, plummeting 628 ft (191 m) in 1 mi (1.6 km). Reach the outlet stream of **Blanca Lake** at 4 mi (6.4 km), 3972 ft (1211 m).

Campsites are clustered near the south shore of the 0.75-mi-long (1.2-km-long) lake. It's possible to continue north, around the lake's west shore, to the snout of Columbia Glacier.

You'd rather not drop to Blanca Lake? Look left (south) near the ridge, before Virgin Lake. A bootbeaten path forks left. It leads south through heather meadows to a sweeping view from atop 5128-ft (1563-m) **Toil Peak**, a wooded bump en route to Troublesome Mtn.

TRIP 40
SPIDER MEADOW / SPIDER GAP

LOCATION	Wenatchee National Forest / Glacier Peak Wilderness
ROUND TRIP	10.4 mi (16.7 km) to lower Spider Meadow
	16.4 mi (26.4 km) to Spider Gap
ELEVATION GAIN	1100 ft (335 m) to meadow, 3600 ft (1097 m) to gap
KEY ELEVATIONS	trailhead 3500 ft (1067 m), meadow 4600 ft (1402 m)
	gap 7100 ft (2164 m)
HIKING TIME	7 to 9 hours for Spider Gap
DIFFICULTY	easy to meadow, challenging to Spider Gap
MAP	*Green Trails* Holden 113

OPINION

The name sounds menacing, but the place is enrapturing. Once you've been to Spider Meadow, its image will serve you as a haven—anytime you're stressed, in need of a restful, comforting thought to restore your calmness and affirm your sanity. Spider Gap has staying power too, but with a very different effect. Whenever you feel jaded, mired in the commonplace, the memory of its harsh, elemental beauty will resuscitate the wildness flickering in your soul.

The forested trail—prettier and more open than the one to nearby Buck Creek Pass—is a pleasant approach. Phelps Creek is audible. The miles pass quickly. You'll soon stride into the spectacle you've anticipated: a vast, sumptuous expanse of greenery bordered by soaring cliffs. Surely this is the Mother of All Meadows. (See inside front cover.)

If you didn't know the trail continued to Spider Gap, you might not believe it possible, and you'd think Spider Meadow was a smashing destination. But it does continue, so you scan the headwall. From here it looks absurdly steep and way too high. Nevertheless, Spider Gap is within striking distance of ambitious, athletic dayhikers.

En route to the gap, Larch Knob is the unlikely location of a marvelous camp—perched high above the valley floor, next to a plunging creek. Behind it is a tremendous gorge beneath the north ridge of Red Mtn and the east end of Chiwawa Mtn. Pouring off the ridge, waterfalls splash over red, rust, orange, and grey rock.

Technically a mere walk-up, the final ascent to the gap might feel too daring for some. If a continuous sense of exposure unnerves you, turn around at Larch Knob, where the trail ends and only a bootbeaten path resumes.

If you're comfortable on sharp ridges, the climactic scramble will thrill you. You'll pass a remnant glacier and tumbling, raw rock, then ascend steep, heathery slopes surrounded by monster peaks. Phelps Basin is 2000 ft (610 m) below.

Approaching the gap, you'll see it's too small and rugged to be called a pass. It's a narrow cleft between Chiwawa and Dumbell mountains. But it does offer ice-axe wielding mountaineers a passage: down Lyman Glacier to Lyman Lakes (Trip 49).

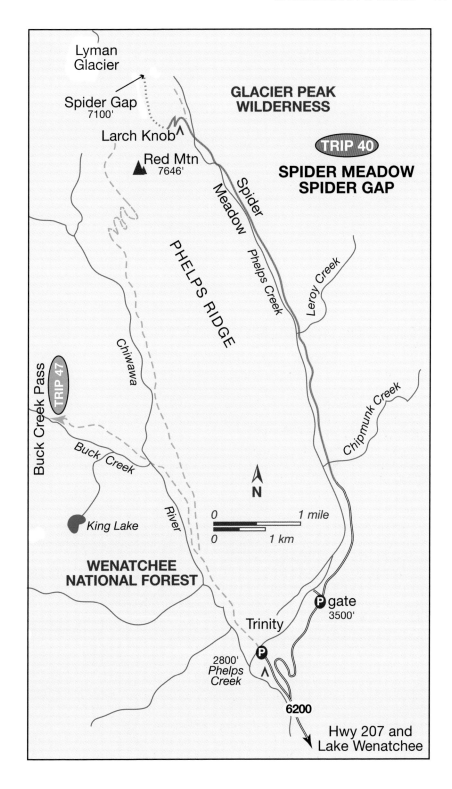

Lyman
Glacier

Spider Gap
7100'

Larch Knob ^

Red Mtn
7646'

GLACIER PEAK
WILDERNESS

TRIP 40

SPIDER MEADOW
SPIDER GAP

Spider Meadow

Phelps Creek

Leroy Creek

PHELPS RIDGE

Chiwawa

Buck Creek Pass

TRIP 47

Buck Creek

Chipmunk Creek

River

King Lake

WENATCHEE
NATIONAL FOREST

N

0   1 mile
0   1 km

P gate
3500'

Trinity

2800'
Phelps
Creek

P

^

6200

Hwy 207 and
Lake Wenatchee

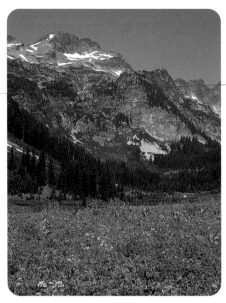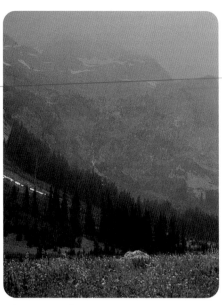

Clear day over Spider Meadow. One hour later a storm moves in.

Hikers with nothing more than trekking poles in hand should turn back from Spider Gap after taking the breakneck plunge north with their eyes only.

FACT

BY VEHICLE

Drive Hwy 2 to Coles Corner, 19.5 mi (31.4 km) east of Stevens Pass, or 16 mi (25.7 km) northwest of Leavenworth. Turn north onto Hwy 207, reset your trip odometer to zero, and proceed toward Lake Wenatchee. Pass the state park and the road to Plain. At 4.3 mi (6.9 km), go right (east) toward the Chiwawa Loop Road. At 5.7 mi (9.2 km) turn left onto Meadow Creek Road, which leads north to Fish Lake and the Chiwawa River valley. Pavement ends at 16.8 mi (27 km). At 28.1 mi (45.2 km) fork right. The road ascends to reach the Phelps Creek trailhead at 30.4 mi (48.9 km), 3500 ft (1067 m). Peaks, snow-fields and waterfalls are visible from the road.

ON FOOT

Follow the abandoned mining road—now a pine-needle-covered path through dense forest—beyond the gate, initially north-northeast. At 0.2 mi (0.3 km) pass a right fork ascending east to Carne Mtn.

The road gradually narrows, heading generally north, following Phelps Creek upstream, above its right (east) bank. Enter Glacier Peak Wilderness and pass a campsite at 2.7 mi (4.3 km). At 3.1 mi (5 km) rockhop a creek and walk through glades.

Reach a treed camp beside a meadow, near Leroy Creek, at 3.5 mi (5.6 km), 4175 ft (1273 m). Cross the creek on a footlog or rockhop it in late summer. Upstream 100 yd (110 m) is a waterfall—welcome refreshment on a hot day. The

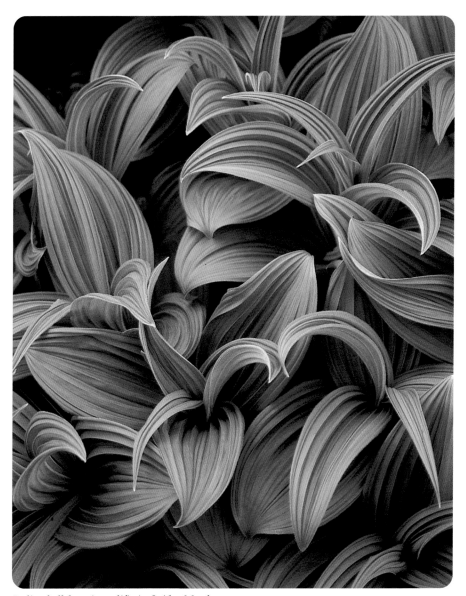

Indian hellebore is prolific in Spider Meadow.

road is now a trail, gently ascending north-northwest toward the upper reaches of Phelps Creek. Cross another bridged tributary at 4.6 mi (7.4 km).

Spider Meadow spreads out before you at 5.2 mi (8.4 km), 4600 ft (1402 m). There are good campsites here, in trees near Phelps Creek. Red Mtn is left (northwest). The meadow is home to a plethora of wildflowers: pinkish-purple asters, tiny bluebells-of-Scotland, pink monkeyflower, the compact white flowers of yarrow, pink steeplebush, columbine, and asters that can be 2 ft (0.6 m) high by early August. Farther along, Indian hellebore dominates.

Commonly known as corn lily, Indian hellebore has long, bright green, accordion-pleated leaves that grow in swirls in early summer. By late summer, numerous, tiny, pale-green flowers appear on the 8 to 10 branches per stalk. Corn lily is extremely poisonous if injested.

The trail steepens near the north end of the meadow. At 6.5 mi (10.5 km), rockhop Phelps Creek where there's an obvious trail on the west bank. Proceed north.

Reach a signed fork and a campsite at 6.7 mi (10.8 km), 5300 ft (1615 m). The Phelps Creek trail continues right, 0.5 mi (0.8 km) north into Phelps Basin. Turn left for Spider Gap and Lyman Lakes. The narrow trail climbs short switchbacks generally west-southwest for 0.4 mi (0.6 km) up a cliff band. It's then a dirt path across a grassy slope.

At 7.5 mi (12.1 km), 6200 ft (1890 m), reach **Larch Knob**—a treed (larches, obviously), rocky peninsula above Spider Meadow and beneath Red Mtn. Sometimes referred to as Spider Glacier camp, it accommodates about four tents. From here, you can survey the entire meadow below. Seven Fingered Jack and Mt. Maude, both over 9000 ft (2743 m), are southeast. A glacier-fed creek rushes past the knob and plunges into the valley.

Beyond Larch Knob is Spider Glacier—now a mere ice-filled couloir sloping 0.75 mi (1.2 km) north up to Spider Gap. It's an easy ascent with an ice axe. When the snow is soft enough for solid footing, some hikers ascend it using only trekking poles. Even if you don't continue that way, walk the first 20 yd/m into the gorge to see the red and orange cliffs of Chiwawa Mtn.

You can also reach Spider Gap by following a rock-and-heather route generally north-northwest along the ridge immediately right (east) of the ice. From Larch Knob, follow the steep, eroded, faint path until it branches, then go whichever way appears safest.

The ice is about 60 yd/m to your left, but you'll soon lose sight of it. Higher now, travel through less heather and more rock. Watch for sporadic cairns. Easy and precarious stretches alternate. Keep to the ridgecrest, away from the cliff. There's one 15-yd/m band of exposed rock to cross. Then the terrain relents. The way is now mostly level, across dirt and rock, toward a looming, dark buttress of Dumbell Mtn. Phelps Creek valley is 2000 ft (610 m) below you.

When you see Spider Gap, the scree slope beneath it might look formidable. It's easier than it appears. Proceed over rock, perhaps on patchy snow, but right of the ice.

Bootbeaten tread leads to 7100-ft (2164-m) **Spider Gap**, 8.2 mi (13.2 km) from the trailhead. Lyman Lakes are visible below (north). Beyond and above them are Cloudy Pass, Cloudy Peak, and North Star Mtn. Sitting Bull Mtn is northwest.

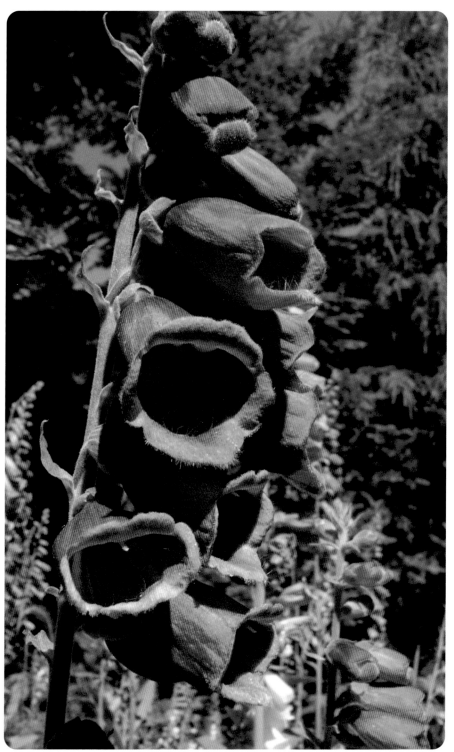

Foxglove thrives along low elevation roadsides.

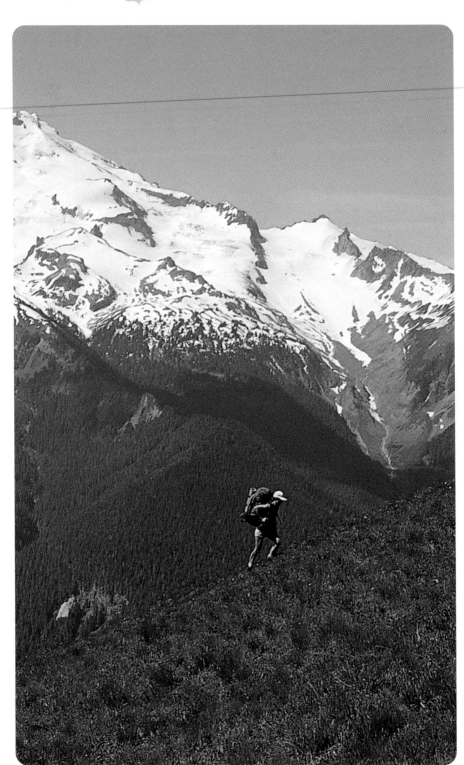

En route to Image Lake (Trip 44), across from Glacier Peak

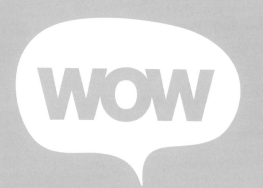

BACKPACK
TRIPS

TRIP 41

HORSESHOE BASIN

LOCATION	Pasayten Wilderness / Okanogan National Forest
ROUND TRIP	13 mi (21 km) for basin, longer for Boundary Trail
ELEVATION GAIN	1200 ft (366 m) to basin, more for Boundary Trail
KEY ELEVATIONS	trailhead 5800 ft (1768 m), Horseshoe Pass 7000 ft (2134 m)
HIKING TIME	2 days for basin, up to 6 days for Boundary Trail
DIFFICULTY	easy
MAPS	*Green Trails* Horseshoe Basin 21, Coleman Peak 20

OPINION

Mountains are vertical. They stand—defiant and forbidding. Meadows are horizontal. They lounge—relaxed and welcoming. Mountains are severe, harsh, rocky. Meadows are serene, soft, carpeted. Mountains, above treeline, are mostly lifeless shades of black, brown and grey, or sterile white. Meadows are vibrantly alive, brilliant green, frequently dappled with psychedelic wildflowers. Mountains sternly demand effort and risk. Meadows kindly invite ease and comfort.

That's why a meadow clutched among mountains is an alluring haven. Why entering a meadow, even one you anticipated thanks to a map or guidebook, feels like a discovery. And why Horseshoe Basin should be high on your *gotta hike* list.

The rolling meadowlands of Horseshoe Basin are extraordinarily vast and remarkably accessible. Most alpine destinations are distant. This one's just 4.5 gently-ascending miles from road's end. High-country trails are usually snow-covered until late July. Here, on the dry east side of the range, consistently sunny skies, and open, sparse forest ensure the trail is hikeable in late June, when the dazzling flower display begins.

Don't even think about dayhiking to Horseshoe Basin. Hoist your backpack and spend at least one night. Reaching this ethereal landscape only to leave immediately would be a wasted effort, because the approach is not scenic. Only beyond where the basin comes into view is this a premier journey. You might want to sit and stare. You might want to explore. Probably both. So allow plenty of time.

The rounded summits will seduce you into roaming higher. Though the views on top are not spectacular, it's liberating to wander at will in such openness. Another temptation is trekking farther west along the Boundary Trail. From Horseshoe Basin, it's 94 mi (151 km) to Harts Pass. Teapot Dome is a satisfying destination for a 3- to 4-day trip. If you push on, the trail clings to the 7000-ft (2134-m) level as far as Cathedral Peak—a good turnaround point for a 5- or 6-day trip. Staying so high for so long is a rare treat in any mountain range. Upper Cathedral Lake, at the base of Amphitheater Mtn's granite cliffs,

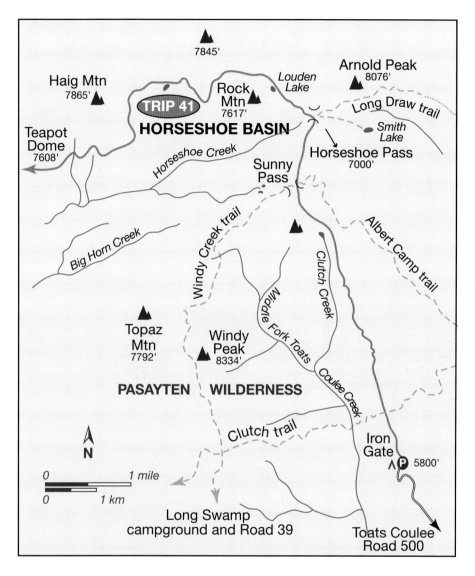

7845'

Haig Mtn
7865'

Teapot
Dome
7608'

TRIP 41

HORSESHOE BASIN

Rock
Mtn
7617'

Louden
Lake

Arnold Peak
8076'

Long Draw trail

Smith
Lake

Horseshoe Pass
7000'

Horseshoe Creek

Sunny
Pass

Big Horn Creek

Windy Creek trail

Middle Fork Toats

Clutch Creek

Albert Camp trail

Topaz
Mtn
7792'

Windy
Peak
8334'

PASAYTEN   WILDERNESS

Coulee Creek

N

0   1 mile
0   1 km

Clutch trail

Iron
Gate
5800'

Long Swamp
campground and Road 39

Toats Coulee
Road 500

is an outstanding destination. Beyond Cathedral Peak the trail skulks in forest
for long periods.

No need to steel yourself for severe ascents and descents. In the 20 mi
(32.2 km) from the basin to Cathedral Peak, the trail loses only a few hundred
feet (100 meters) in a couple places, and it gains only 1000 ft (305 m) over
Apex Pass. So you can relax and enjoy. Just go as far as you feel compelled,
then camp wherever you want (with minimal impact, of course). Permits,
reservations and rigid itineraries are not required here in the Pasayten Wilderness, as they are in the national park.

The initial 4 mi (6.4 km) through scrawny lodgepole pines can be
discouraging. Just press on. You'll soon burst into tundra meadows more like
the Scottish Highlands than the craggy Cascades. Luscious fields of lavender
lupine and bright-yellow subalpine buttercup blanket the slopes. A closer

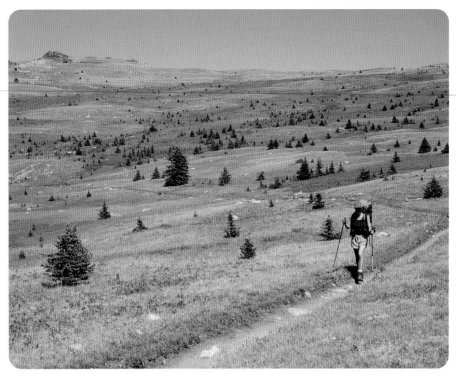

Horseshoe Basin

look will reveal velvety, pink-plumed avens, and magenta shooting stars. Of course, you'll also see the ubiquitous, red Indian paintbrush.

Too bad the mosquitoes are so horrendous. Otherwise you could lollygag in the meadows. Given enough time in such a halcyon atmosphere, you might learn aromatherapy from the flowers or maybe even levitation from the cottonball clouds. But the reality is, without a steady, stiff breeze to keep the bloodsuckers down, it can be difficult to sit outside your tent for long. At least rain is unlikely here, so you can probably leave the fly off your tent.

On the north side of Rock Mtn, a mile past Horseshoe Pass, you'll exit the meadows and enter dry, sparse, airy forest offering occasional open views. Dusty trail gives way to crushed gravel—very pleasant. Your eye is drawn to twisted, silver deadfall, instead of sweeping tundra. Granite slabs and outcroppings give the land sharper edges. From here on, it's not a particular scenic feature that pulls you on, but rather your emotions, evoked by the expansive environment. You might notice a peaceful buoyancy stealing over you—very different from the solemnity you perhaps experience in a deep valley, or the exhilaration you probably feel on a mountaintop.

Mountain bikes are not permitted in this fragile area. Riding all the way to Cathedral Peak in a day would be a thrill, but you can get an adrenalin rush lots of other places. Horseshoe Basin deserves to be appreciated more fully.

There's no creek at the trailhead, and the region is arid, so bring plenty of water in your vehicle—enough so you can start the trip with full bottles. Refill at every opportunity along the trail.

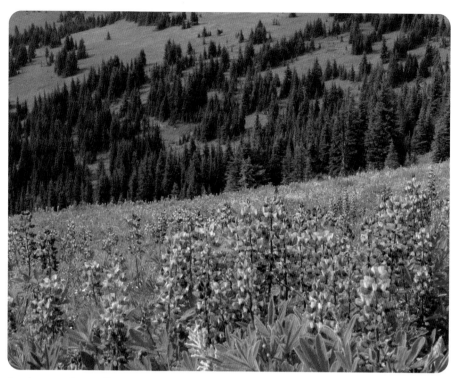

Lupine near Sunny Pass

FACT

BY VEHICLE

From British Columbia, drive Hwy 3 into Washington. Enter the U.S. at the Chopaka-Nighthawk border crossing, then continue south to Loomis.

From within Washington, drive Hwy 97 north to Ellisforde, then proceed 12 mi (19.3 km) northwest to Loomis.

From either approach, drive 0.3 mi (0.5 km) through Loomis to the signed T-intersection. Go right 1.9 mi (3.1 km) to Toats Coulee Road 39 and turn left onto it near the valley bottom, before the highway turns sharply right. Reset your trip odometer to zero. At 1.3 mi (2.1 km) proceed straight on pavement, ignoring the ascending dirt road. At 7.9 mi (12.7 km) go left at the signed junction. Pass North Fork campground on the right at 8.2 mi (13.2 km). Reach a junction at 13.7 mi (22 km). Turn right (northwest) onto Road (3900) 500. Reach Iron Gate campground and the trailhead parking area at 19.7 mi (31.7 km), 5800 ft (1768 m).

ON FOOT

The trail, initially an abandoned mining road, leads north. At 0.7 mi (1.1 km) proceed straight at a junction. About 20 yd/m farther is another junction. Again continue straight. Your general direction of travel will remain north-northwest all the way to Sunny Pass.

At 3 mi (4.8 km) enter an open area of grass and flowers, then re-enter trees. After a steep stretch, the trail leaves the lodgepole pines at 4.5 mi (7.2 km). Cross a creeklet and arrive in **Sunny Basin**. You'll find treed tentsites here, east of the trail, beside a small creek, at 6900 ft (2103 m). Beyond, the trail plies grass and flowers to Horseshoe Basin and most of the 6 mi (9.7 km) to Haig Mtn.

At 5.2 mi (8.4 km) reach 7200-ft (2195-m) **Sunny Pass**. The ragged summit of 8685-ft (2647-m) Remmel Mtn is visible southwest. Your immediate goal—Horseshoe Basin—is also in view, as are the tame, grassy peaks above it: Rock Mtn (north-northwest), and Arnold Peak (north-northeast).

Bear right at Sunny Pass, ignoring the multi-track trail forking left and heading southwest to Windy Peak. Just 180 yd (200 m) farther, bear left and follow the main trail north.

Horseshoe Pass is at 6.5 mi (10.5 km), 7000 ft (2134 m). If the seasonal creek here is dry, the right spur leads 0.8 mi (1.3 km) east to Smith Lake, but that too can evaporate in late summer. To continue on the Boundary Trail, bear left (northwest) from Horseshoe Pass. Reach **Louden Lake** at 7.5 mi (12.1 km). Though it can disappear as well, you'll find comfortable campsites above its southwest shore.

At 7.7 mi (12.4 km), near the northeast edge of **Rock Mtn**, a right spur leads north to appealing campsites in meadows among larch and whitebark pines. The main trail continues west though open forest and low shrubs. Boulders and flowers adorn the hillsides.

A pond is immediately south of the trail at 10 mi (16.1 km). An otherwise inviting campsite, it can be infested with mosquitoes. You might evade them 2.2 mi (3.5 km) farther, on the breezier, open slopes south of **Haig Mtn**. There's a seasonal creeklet there, and a view southeast to Windy Peak, but level ground is scarce.

Gain and lose 100 ft (30 m) a couple times between Horseshoe Basin and the south side of Haig Mtn. The elevation varies from 6900 to 7200 ft (2103 to 2195 m). The trail then drops 320 ft (97.5 m) in 2.5 mi (4 km) to **Teapot Dome**, which is 8 mi (12.9 km) west of Horseshoe Pass, 14.5 mi (23.3 km) from the trailhead. Beneath the dome's southeast wall you'll find granite outcroppings, boulders, the silver skeletons of fallen trees, a seasonal creeklet, and level tentsites.

The terrain beyond Teapot Dome is similar to what you will already have traversed between Rock and Haig mountains. The easy-to-follow Boundary Trail has only one junction, 6.6 mi (10.6 km) after Teapot Dome, where trail 534 descends southeast along Tungsten Creek. Continue straight (northwest) for Cathedral Pass, gaining 1000 ft (305 m) to **Apex Pass** en route.

The trail crosses creeks occasionally, but some are unreliable in late summer. Fill water bottles whenever possible. Reach 7600-ft (2316-m) **Cathedral Pass** at 26 mi (41.8 km), immediately below 8601-ft (2622-m) Cathedral Peak (right/north). **Upper Cathedral Lake** is 0.7 mi (1.1 km) farther—below and southwest of the pass, at the base of Amphitheater Mtn's granite walls.

COPPER RIDGE / WHATCOM PASS

LOCATION	Mt. Baker Wilderness / North Cascades National Park
CIRCUIT	45 mi (72.4 km)
ELEVATION GAIN	10,000 ft (3048 m)
KEY ELEVATIONS	trailhead 3100 ft (945 m), Hannegan Pass 5100 ft (1555 m)
	Copper Ridge lookout 6260 ft (1908 m)
	Chilliwack River 2200 ft (671 m)
	Whatcom Pass 5206 ft (1587 m)
HIKING TIME	5 days
DIFFICULTY	challenging
MAPS	*Green Trails* Mt. Shuksan 14, Mt. Challenger 15

OPINION

Want to add a coveted merit badge to your ceremonial hiking tunic?

Test your mettle here, on a grand circuit over Hannegan Pass, across Copper Ridge, along the Chilliwack River, and up to Whatcom Pass near the Challenger Glacier.

The river valley is deep and dark, the trees ancient and huge, the ridge long and panoramic, the peaks towering and icy, the tranquility pervasive and divine.

So too, the flies are innumerable and pestiferous, the deadfall frequent and immense, the brush riotous and cloying, the ascents long and severe.

It's a true journey. A five-day trek. By the effete standards of our pampered culture, it's positively Homeric. Yet it's achievable and enjoyable for any moderately experienced, reasonably fit backpacker.

Your odyssey begins in Ruth Creek valley. Cliffs, waterfalls, avalanche greenery and snowfields will stoke your enthusiasm on the easy walk to Hannegan Pass. You then plunge past the colorful soils of ancient volcanoes into the headwater drainage of the Chilliwack River, beneath Ruth Mtn. From there, you'll vault onto Copper Ridge.

Here, the trail rides the sky, offering a string of vistas that rival any in the range, culminating with the closest view that non-climbers can attain of Mount Redoubt. The intricacies of the ridge itself are fascinating too. Copper Lake sits in a classic alpine cirque. The trail wiggles through fields of rectangular boulders, some resembling beds and chaise lounges, that entice you to drop your pack and sprawl.

Then the good times are over, temporarily, on the abrupt descent into the Chilliwack River Valley. With your body feeling like a runaway train, either your trekking poles or your knees will take the brunt of this 4-mi (6.4-km), 3560-ft (1055-m) drop.

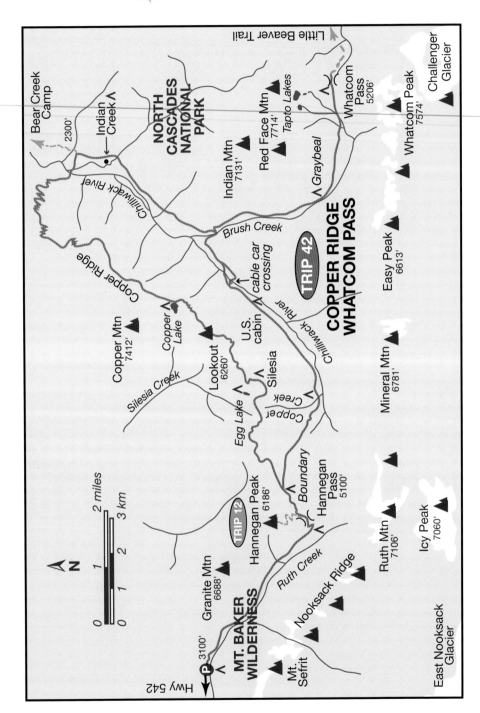

COPPER RIDGE
WHATCOM PASS

TRIP 42

TRIP 12

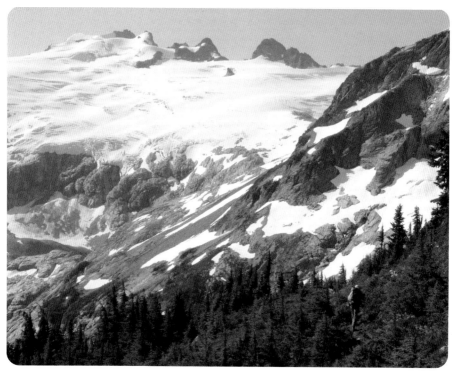

Challenger Glacier, from just above Whatcom Pass

After fording the braided Chilliwack River, you face 8.7 mi (14 km) of alternating overgrown trail and viewless forest en route to Whatcom Pass, where you'll confront the Challenger Glacier. Suddenly, your tribulations will seem minor—especially if you veer off the main trail to superior viewpoints on either side. Tapto Lakes, north of and above the pass, is the supreme vantage.

Tapto is also the most desirable place to pitch your tent on the entire circuit, though Whatcom camp, in the pass, is no ghetto. Another option is to dayhike up to the pass from a basecamp at flood-damaged but serviceable Graybeal, which *is* a ghetto of fallen trees.

All the campgrounds are small. Each has only a few tentsites, reducing the chance you'll be irritated by the neighbors. Hannegan camp, a mere 5 mi (8 km) from the trailhead, is the only one not in the national park. All the others require a permit.

To make backcountry camping reservations, stop at a national park office in person the day before your trip. If you wait until the morning of, you'll be less likely to secure the sites you want. For details, read about *Backcountry Permits* in the introduction of this book.

Presuming you can start reasonably early on day one, and you want to spend as much time as possible on Copper Ridge and at Whatcom Pass, here's the optimal itinerary for a five day, four night, clockwise circuit: (1) Silesia camp/Egg Lake or Copper Lake, (2) Indian Creek, (3) Whatcom camp or Tapto Lakes, (4) U.S. Cabin camp.

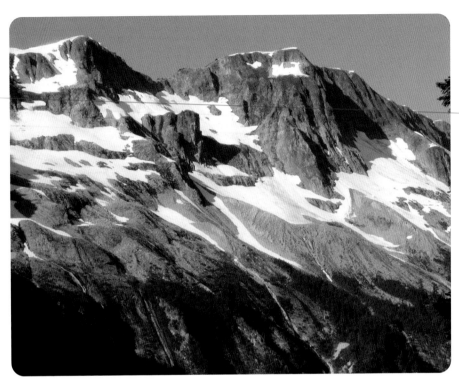

Whatcom Peak, from just above Graybeal camp

Of course, you have options other than the full, five-day circuit. A three-day trip, for example, will allow you to appreciate one of the two scenic climaxes.

If you're going to Copper Ridge but not Whatcom Pass, don't hike a circuit. Go out and back along the ridge, enjoying the tremendous views twice, rather than enduring the steep descent into the Chilliwack River Valley and the long, viewless march back out of it.

If you're going to Whatcom Pass but not Copper Ridge, consider staying two nights at U.S. Cabin camp and dayhiking from there to the pass. U.S. Cabin is beautiful, and though it's farther from the pass than Graybeal is, you'll enjoy your campsite more, you'll carry a full pack for a shorter distance, and you'll be positioned for an easier hike all the way out on day three.

Bear in mind, U.S. Cabin is in ancient forest, beside the Chilliwack River. It's dark but soothing. Whatcom camp is among mountain hemlocks in the subalpine zone. It's protected but has quick access to impressive scenery. Tapto Lakes is above treeline. It's exposed but spectacular. Each is distinctly different. You might prefer the higher-elevation camps, despite having to haul your full pack all the way up and back.

Given only three days, we'd choose Copper Ridge over Whatcom Pass. Whatcom Peak and the Challenger Glacier are visible from the ridge, plus you'll see infinitely more. An out-and-back ridgewalk greatly reduces the time you'll spend in forest. Whatcom Pass is itself just below treeline, as is the hike to and from. Still, the five-day circuit described below is best. We once hiked

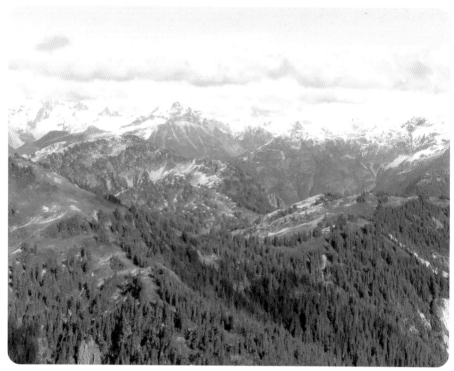

Copper Ridge, from Hannegan Peak

the ridge but skipped the pass due to inclement weather. Not seeing it tormented us until we could return, years later.

When should you start this adventure?

Steep, rugged stretches of Copper Ridge typically hold snow until late July. Go earlier only if you're equipped to safely travel through snow, or the park service has assured you the ridge is snow free. September is when the area's notorious fly infestation subsides and when you're most likely to get five days of good weather.

Always desirable on a backpack trip, good weather is a requirement here. Adjust your plans according to the long-range forecast. If the clouds are low and rain persists, you'll see little but trees. And you'll get soaked to the skin, regardless of what miracle barrier fabric you're wearing, because you'll probably plow through long stretches of dense brush. Wet brush = wet hiker. Meager budgets make trail crews increasingly scarce, so it's doubtful one will have preceded you. Expect brush.

The brush you'll encounter will surely be rife with stinging nettles, too. So you'll want long pants and a long-sleeve shirt. On our last trip here, we decided the vegetation must be carnivorous, it had so many fangs and claws. Even if you're lucky, and the trail's been recently brushed, sleeves and pants will help safeguard your sanity when you're besieged by flies.

FACT

BY VEHICLE

From the Glacier Public Service Center on Highway 542, drive east 13.1 mi (21.1 km). Just before the Nooksack River bridge, turn left (east) onto Road 32 toward Hannegan Pass. At the junction in 1.3 mi (2.1 km), stay left on Ruth Creek Road 32. At 5.4 mi (8.7 km) reach the road's end campground and trailhead, at 3100 ft (945 m). On weekends, expect to see dozens of vehicles here. The tentsites are between the parking lot and Ruth Creek.

ON FOOT

The trail is initially level. It leads east, gradually curving southeast, following Ruth Creek upstream.

Within ten minutes, the steep cliffs of Mt. Sefrit and Nooksack Ridge are visible right (south) across the valley. Continue through beautiful, mature, mountain-hemlock forest with occasional views.

At 3 mi (5 km), 4000 ft (1220 m) the ascent begins in earnest. About 1½ hours from the trailhead, a right spur drops to a creeklet then rises to **Hannegan camp** on a knoll. Visible south is glacier dolloped, 7106-ft (2166-m) Ruth Mtn. The main trail begins a switchbacking ascent generally north.

Fifteen minutes above the campground, enter 5100-ft (1555-m) **Hannegan Pass** at 4 mi (6.4 km) and reach a junction. Left ascends north 1 mi (1.6 km) to Hannegan Peak. Right is a climbers' route curving south toward Ruth Mtn. Proceed straight on the main trail, contouring briefly before switchbacking generally east, down into the headwater drainage of the Chilliwack River.

After descending 500 ft (152 m) in 0.7 mi (1.1 km), hop over a creek and cross a rockslide. The white talus and greyish clay slope on the right (south) is an arm of Ruth Mtn. Colorful, striated soil distinguishes the slopes to the left (north).

Enter North Cascades National Park and reach a fork at 5 mi (8 km), 4400 ft (1341 m). Straight continues east, immediately passes **Boundary camp**, then curves southeast, diving deeper into the Chilliwack River Valley—your return route on this grand circuit. Turn left and begin ascending northeast to Copper Ridge.

Boundary camp is on the right, in subalpine forest, next to a corn-lily meadow, above the Chilliwack River, which at this early stage is merely a creek. The tentsites are just inside the national park, so a camping permit is necessary.

Ascending to Copper Ridge, at 6 mi (9.7 km) attain a view southwest back to Hannegan Pass and south to the enormous wall of 7060-ft (2152-m) Icy Peak. Traverse the top of Hells Gorge at 6.7 mi (10.8 km), 5400 ft (1646 m). Just beyond, enter heather meadows at the **southwest end of Copper Ridge**. The Silesia Creek valley is far below (north). Beyond it are the Border Peaks.

The trail undulates generally east along the knobby ridge to **Silesia camp** at 8.2 mi (13.2 km), 5689 ft (1734 m). There are only two tent sites here. The views southeast to Mineral Mountain and Easy Ridge are exceptional. Below Silesia, a left spur drops 300 ft (91 m) northwest to **Egg Lake** and three more tent sites. The lake is the immediate area's only reliable water source.

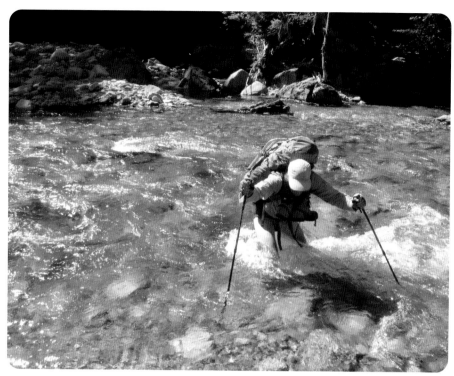

Learning why the cable car near U.S. Cabin camp is preferable to fording the Chilliwack River

Continuing northeast along the ridge, the trail drops 280 ft (85 m) then ascends 1100 ft (335 m) on tight switchbacks to **Copper Ridge lookout** at 10.2 mi (16.4 km), 6260 ft (1910 m). A ranger resides here during the summer hiking season.

To the southwest, Ruth Mtn, Icy Peak, Mt. Shuksan, and Mt. Baker are visible. Mt. Blum is directly south. Southeast across the Chilliwack River Valley is the Picket Range massif, including Whatcom Peak and Mt. Challenger.

From the small summit where the lookout is perched, the trail proceeds northeast, descending 250 ft (76 m). The views continue, with Bear Mtn and Mt. Redoubt visible northeast. After contouring 0.5 mi (0.8 km), the trail makes a steep, rugged descent to a three-site camp near vivid-blue **Copper Lake** at 11.4 mi (18.4 km), 5200 ft (1585 m).

Soon rockhop across a tumbling creek. At 12.2 mi (19.6 km) pass through a boulder garden, then gear down for the last ascent on the ridge. After gaining 400 ft (122 m) via steep switchbacks, the trail regains the ridgecrest near 5760 ft (1756 m) and offers a view directly south up Brush Creek—the way to Whatcom Pass. Farther north on Copper Ridge, the eastern horizon is dominated by 8956-ft (2730-m) Mount Redoubt. You can also survey the Indian Creek valley on the south side of Bear Mtn. During this final ridge run, the trail contours 1.5 mi (2.4 km) through heather meadows.

Before the trail plummets east off the **northeast end of Copper Ridge**, Chilliwack Lake makes a surprise appearance north, far below. At 14.5 mi (23.3 km) the trail drops steeply below a cliff and a long-lingering snowfield, then darts upward to skirt a rockslide. Descending again, it leads farther north than seems necessary. Be patient and observant. The trail is rooty and at times is a narrow trench—awkward to stay in without tripping. Rocks on the path might be hidden by tall grass. The trail then traverses the top of another rockslide before fully committing to the long, forested plunge to the Chilliwack River.

Cross a reliable spring and a stream at 15.4 mi (24.8 km). Nearing the valley bottom at 18.3 mi (29.5 km) the trail is faint. Cairns and flagging direct you across the **Chilliwack River** ford at 2200 ft (670 m). By September, the river's main branch should be less than knee deep and only about 25 ft (8 m) wide, but there might be other branches, including a tributary—Indian Creek. On the far bank, proceed east-southeast 0.25 mi (0.4 km) to intersect the **Chilliwack trail** at 18.9 mi (30.4 km), 2300 ft (701 m).

Left follows the river downstream into Canada. The unmaintained trail is sure to be brushy and riddled with deadfall. For Whatcom Pass and Hannegan trailhead, turn right and hike south. Reach **Indian Creek camp** at 19.7 mi (32 km). It has three sites and room for a couple more tents beneath giant cedars.

Continuing south, cross bridged Indian Creek just after the camp. The trail then heads south-southwest, up the Chilliwack River Valley, but it doesn't stay near the river. At 22.4 mi (36.1 km), 2600 ft (793 m), reach **Brush Creek junction**. Right crosses the bridged creek and continues 12.1 mi (19.5 km) to Hannegan trailhead. Left follows Brush Creek upstream: south 2.2 mi (3.5 km) to Graybeal camp, then east 3 mi (4.8 km) to Whatcom Pass.

Heading to Whatcom Pass, the trail ascends briefly then is mostly level through an ancient fir-and-cedar forest. Unless a trail crew has preceded you, expect brush. About 30 minutes from the junction, follow cairns and flagging through a flood-ravaged area where you'll probably have to rockhop or ford unbridged stream channels. If it's a hot day, might as well dunk yourself in a pool once your boots are off.

Trail resumes beyond the short washed-out stretch. Another 30 minutes of hiking will bring you to **Graybeal camp**, on the right, at 3230 ft (985 m). Previously deluged by floods, the camp is strewn with deadfall. One tentsite at the southwest corner, near the creek bank, affords a view south to Easy Peak.

Beyond Graybeal, the trail ascends steeply. Notice the painstaking trail construction completed many years ago. The logs they used to create secure walkways are still supportive. But other sections desperately need repair. Trails like this are a priceless resource, but if not continually reclaimed, they'll be lost. On your way home, write a note to the national park superintendent requesting trail maintenance, then drop it at the Glacier Public Service Center.

Within 25 minutes, Easy Ridge is visible south through the trees, across Brush Creek canyon. Hop over several creeklets. Thimbleberry, salmonberry, and stinging nettle are profuse. So are wildflowers, including fleabane, spirea, tiger lilies, and bleeding hearts.

At 4000 ft (1220 m), about 45 minutes after departing Graybeal, attain a view south-southeast to nearby Whatcom Peak. In early summer, we counted sixteen cascades flowing off Easy Ridge, west of the peak. The trail continues ascending among ancient trees.

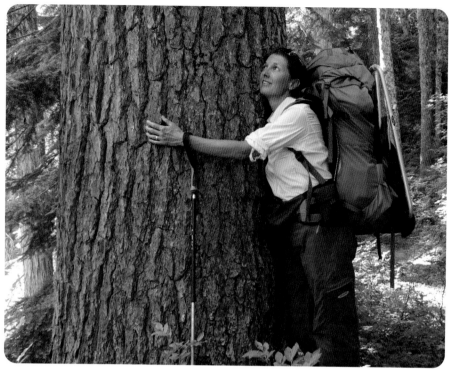

Ancient Douglas fir thrive in the Chilliwack River Valley.

Cross Tapto Creek about one hour above Graybeal. The well-engineered trail—sporadically supported by boulders and lined with rocks—continues ascending. At 5070 ft (1545 m), about two hours above Graybeal, follow a boardwalk through subalpine meadows flanked by mountain hemlocks.

Nearing the pass, hop over a stream where a left (west) spur leads to three tentsites at **Whatcom camp**. A few minutes farther, having hiked 5.2 mi (8.4 km) from Brush Creek junction near the Chilliwack River, and having ascended nearly 2000 ft (610 m) from Graybeal, reach 5206-ft (1587-m) **Whatcom Pass**.

Visible directly south is 7574-ft (2309-m) Whatcom Peak. Southeast is 8236-ft (2510-m) Mt. Challenger, above the Challenger Glacier. Just a few steps beyond where the trail tops out, it nosedives into Little Beaver Creek Valley. Stillwell camp is far below, 6.3 mi (10.1 km) east-northeast.

To better appreciate the dramatic scenery above, follow the right spur south. Your perspective of the glacier will improve significantly within 0.25 mi (0.4 km). Continue ascending to at least 5380 ft (1640 m) before returning to the main trail in the pass.

To survey the area from an even more impressive setting, follow the left spur north-northeast. The way is steep and rough, ascending over a 6000-ft (1829-m) ridge, then dropping to the **Tapto Lakes** at 5740 ft (1750 m), in a small basin beneath Red Face Mtn, about 1 mi (1.6 km) from Whatcom Pass. Cross-country camping is allowed at Tapto, but a permit is required, just as it is for any national-park backcountry campground. The tiny **Middle Lakes**, 1 mi (1.6 km) east-northeast of Tapto, are also hiker accessible.

Upon returning to **Brush Creek junction** from Whatcom Pass, your total hiking distance will be 32.8 mi (52.8 km), not including your explorations above the pass. Heading for Hannegan trailhead now, descend to the bridge spanning Brush Creek. Cross to the west bank and follow the trail north-northwest. It soon curves left (southwest). Proceed through intermittent stands of ancient forest.

Reach a fork at 33.6 mi (54.1 km). Right descends to the Chilliwack River horse ford. Bear left, and at 34.3 mi (55.2 km), 2520 ft (768 m) reach the **cable-car crossing**—a much safer alternative for hikers. Per-person, it takes less energy to propel the car if two hikers squeeze in together.

Above the northwest bank, the trail resumes southwest through what can be a very brushy stretch if a trail crew hasn't preceded you. At 34.8 mi, (56 km), 2640 ft (805 m), about 20 minutes from the cable car, a left spur descends south to **U.S. Cabin camp**: three tentsites beneath ancient cedars, near the river.

Continuing southwest, the main trail is virtually level for 2 mi (3.2 km). After a gentle westward ascent, reach **Copper Creek camp** at 37.4 mi (60.2 km), 3120 ft (950 m). Tentsites here are above the creek's east and west banks, in a forest of Douglas fir, cedar, and mountain hemlock.

The ascent steepens past Copper Creek. Climbing generally west-northwest out of the Chilliwack River Valley, gain 1200 ft (366 m) in the next 2.5 mi (4 km). Just past **Boundary camp**, intersect the Copper Ridge trail at 39.9 mi (64.2 km), 4400 ft (1341 m).

You're now on familiar ground. Right ascends northeast to Copper Ridge. Proceed straight, ascend southwest over **Hannegan Pass**, then descend northwest to **Hannegan traihead**. Upon reaching the parking lot, you'll have hiked more than 45 mi (72.4 km) and ascended approximately 10,000 ft (3048 m).

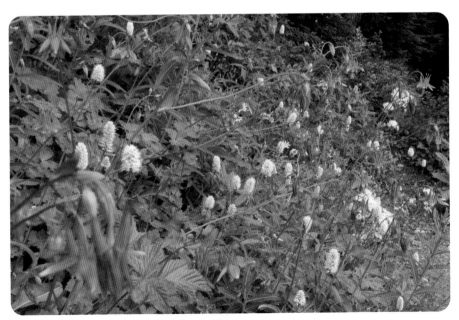

Columbine along Ruth Creek valley trail

PARK CREEK PASS

LOCATION	Ross Lake National Recreation Area
	North Cascades National Park
SHUTTLE TRIP	40.1 mi (64.5 km)
ELEVATION GAIN	8840 ft (2694 m)
KEY ELEVATIONS	Colonial Creek trailhead 1200 ft (366 m)
	Park Creek Pass 6100 ft (1860 m)
	Park Creek camp 2300 ft (701 m)
	Cascade Pass 5400 ft (1646 m)
	Cascade Pass trailhead 3600 ft (1097 m)
HIKING TIME	4 to 5 days
DIFFICULTY	challenging
MAPS	*Green Trails* Diablo Dam 48, Mt. Logan 49
	Cascade Pass 80, McGregor Mtn 81

Thunder *Creek*? Elsewhere in the world, the notion that such a swift, voluminous, bridge-eating torrent is a mere creek would be laughable. But not in the North Cascades. Here, nature is big. Big creeks. Big trees. Even big fungi. And certainly big mountains, often requiring a big journey like this to fully appreciate them.

Start by hiking the entire length of Thunder Creek, from where it ends at Diablo Lake to where it begins high among the peaks. En route, spend an entire day amid giants: fir, cedar, and hemlock. After appreciating and persevering many of the wonders and obstacles peculiar to this great range, top out at Park Creek Pass.

For some, the pass is the destination of a round trip. For others, it's the first of two scenic climaxes on a one-way shuttle trip. Either way, upon arrival you'll likely feel alternating waves of awe and relief.

Pull up a rock. Toast your accomplishment. Marvel at sights above and below. Park Creek Pass is 0.2 mi (0.3 km) long. It's a narrow gap separating the boulder-strewn north side from the meadow-laced south side. Allow time to roam. If this is your turnaround point, devote at least a full day to scrambling higher, perhaps onto the slopes of Buckner Mtn. A single blue-sky summer day of high-elevation romping up here is apt to rank among your most memorable mountain experiences ever.

Camping is prohibited at the pass, so pitch your tent beneath the north side, in Thunder Basin. If proceeding through the pass, spend the next night beneath the south side, at Buckner camp. From there, continue down to the Stehekin Valley where you have two shuttle-trip options of similar length: (1) Left to Bridge Creek, then out the Pacific Crest Trail to Hwy 20 near Rainy Pass, or (2) Right to Cottonwood camp, then up to Pelton Basin, over Cascade Pass, and down to the Cascade River Road.

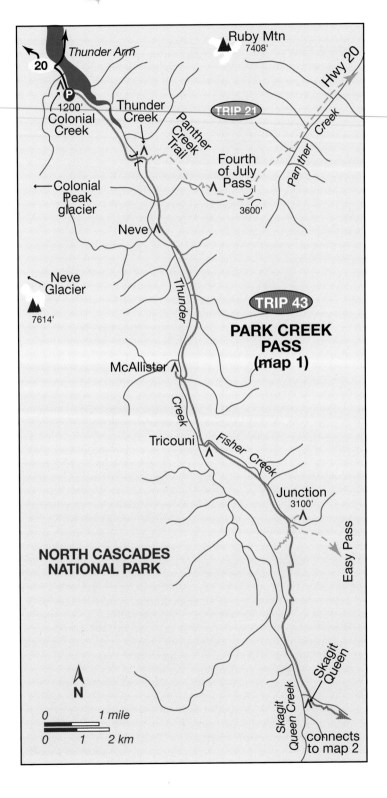

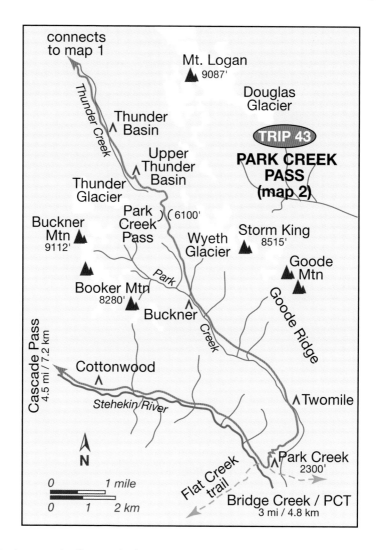

connects to map 1

Mt. Logan
▲ 9087'

Douglas Glacier

Thunder Creek

Thunder Basin

Upper Thunder Basin

TRIP 43
PARK CREEK PASS
(map 2)

Thunder Glacier

Park Creek Pass

(6100'

Wyeth Glacier

Storm King
8515'

Buckner Mtn ▲
9112'

Goode Mtn ▲

Park

Booker Mtn
8280' ▲

Buckner

Goode Ridge

Cascade Pass
4.5 mi / 7.2 km

Cottonwood

Creek

Stehekin River

Twomile

N

Park Creek
2300'

0   1 mile

0   1   2 km

Flat Creek trail

Bridge Creek / PCT
3 mi / 4.8 km

Option one is disappointing, monotonous, a scenic zero. It allows for an easier shuttle arrangement or hitchhike between trailheads, but in every other respect option two is superior. After completing the Park Creek Pass / Cascade Pass through-trip, if you must hitchhike, it shouldn't be difficult. Enough people dayhike to Cascade Pass that snagging a ride from the trailhead down to Marblemount is simply a matter of asking. You'll then be on Hwy 20, where lots of cars will be heading toward Colonial Creek campground and can drop you near your vehicle.

No, it's not the transport between trailheads that should concern you. It's the challenges you'll face along the trail.

The long march to Park Creek Pass will test your patience by granting you only an occasional skyward view. It's like a swimming-pool bully who keeps dunking your head under water. Try to simply enjoy the lush, ancient forest en route. The pass is sublime, but it's distant, deeply embedded in the South Unit of North Cascades National Park.

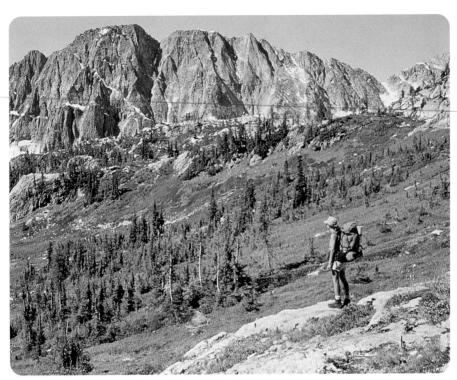

Booker Mountain, from south side of Park Creek Pass

Also beware the 3 B's: bears, bugs, brush. This is one of the few places we've seen bears in the North Cascades. They were black bears, not grizzlies. They were skittish and posed no threat. But they were bears nonetheless. We've also seen more bear scat here than elsewhere in the range. The bruins probably won't bother you, but their obvious presence might keep you on edge. The Cascades' notorious biting flies *will* bother you in midsummer. Only at the pass might you escape them. As for brush, expect nettles the last couple miles before Thunder Basin, thick alder on the descent south of the pass, and a veritable jungle on other stretches that haven't been recently cleared by a trail crew.

Continuing south from the pass, you'll drop below treeline into the Park Creek drainage. It's anticlimactic. You've been booted out of heaven, back to earth. The forest is drier and less impressive here than in the Thunder Creek drainage. But if you're heading for Cascade Pass—especially if you've never dayhiked there—you can look forward to a spectacular end to this supreme trek through the lonely depths of North Cascades National Park.

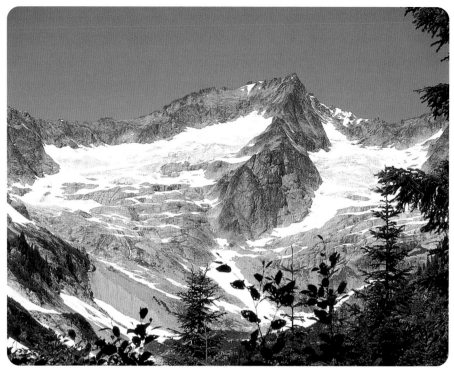

Buckner Mountain, from just north of Park Creek Pass

FACT

BY VEHICLE

For the one-way shuttle trip described below, the starting and ending trailheads are both off Hwy 20. You'll begin hiking south of Diablo Lake. You'll finish hiking at the Cascade River Road, south of Marblemount. Here's how to reach those two trailheads.

From the Diablo-townsite turnoff, drive Hwy 20 southeast 4.3 mi (6.9 km) to Colonial Creek campground on Diablo Lake. Turn southeast into the big parking lot, then proceed through the campground to the smaller parking lot at the trailhead. **The hike begins here**, at 1200 ft (366 m).

At the east edge of Marblemount, where Hwy 20 bends north, go straight (east) onto Cascade River Road and immediately cross the Skagit River. At 0.7 mi (1.1 km) pass the Rockport-Cascade Road on the right. Continue east on Cascade River Road 15. Pavement ends at 5.2 mi (8.4 km). At 8.3 mi (13.4 km) pass the entrance to Marble Creek campground. At 16.9 mi (27.2 km) curve sharply left, ignoring a right fork to the Cascade River trails. Enter the national park at 18.3 mi (29.5 km). At 23.5 mi (37.8 km) the road ends in the spacious Cascade Pass trailhead parking lot. **The hike ends here**, at 3600 ft (1097 m).

Before setting out, it's helpful to have the following figures in mind. It's 19.8 mi (31.9 km) to Park Creek Pass, 7.2 mi (11.6 km) from there to Stehekin Valley, 9.4 mi (15.1 km) from there to Cascade Pass, and 3.7 mi (6 km) from there to the Cascade River Road. You'll ascend 5740 ft (1750 m) to Park Creek Pass, and 3100 ft (945 m) from Stehekin Valley to Cascade Pass.

Ready? Let's go. The trail leads southeast, along the west shore of Diablo Lake's Thunder Arm. Ignore the signed nature trail. Proceed upstream along the west bank of Thunder Creek.

About 30 minutes from the trailhead, cross a bridge to the creek's east bank, pass **Thunder Creek camp**, and reach a signed junction at 2 mi (3.2 km). Left ascends to Fourth of July Pass. Go right and continue following Thunder Creek upstream generally south.

Neve camp is in big timber, on the right, at 2.5 mi (4 km). At 6.8 mi (10.9 km), 1900 ft (579 m) a right spur crosses to Thunder Creek's west bank then heads north 0.5 mi (0.8 km) to tentsites near McAllister Creek. At 7.2 mi (11.6 km) enter North Cascades National Park.

Cross the Fisher Creek bridge at 8.1 mi (13 km), 2000 ft (610 m) and arrive at **Tricouni camp**. To avoid the largest swampland in the Cascades, the trail veers left and soon begins a 1100-ft (335-m) ascent southeast to **Junction camp** at 10.3 mi (16.6 km), 3100 ft (945 m).

En route to Park Creek Pass, this is the only campground with views. Tricouni and Primus peaks (west, across the canyon) and the upper reaches of Thunder Creek are visible. Tentsites here are on both sides of the trail.

At Junction camp, ignore the Fisher Creek trail forking left. It leads 14.8 mi (23.8 km) generally east, over Easy Pass, to Hwy 20. The trail to Park Creek Pass continues south.

At 10.5 mi (16.9 km) ignore a right spur descending sharply southwest. The main trail gradually descends south to 2260 ft (690 m)—a frustrating loss of 840 ft (256 m). Your compensation is a fine view of Boston Glacier (south).

Pursuing the relinquished elevation, the trail climbs to a bridged crossing of Thunder Creek and, immediately after, a fork at 14.1 mi (22.7 km), 3100 ft (945 m). Right is a 0.2-mi (0.3-km) spur dropping to **Skagit Queen camp**, near Skagit Queen Creek. The main trail ascends left (east-southeast), still following Thunder Creek upstream.

Gain 900 ft (274 m) in 1.2 mi (1.9 km), passing huge moss-covered boulders, to enter a hanging valley near 15.3 mi (24.6 km), 4000 ft (1219 m), beneath Mt. Logan.

Heading southeast, attain your first glimpse of Park Creek Pass. Though it appears close, it's still about two hours distant. Ford Thunder Creek to its left (northeast) bank near Thunder Basin Stock camp and continue following the now diminished creek upstream.

At the first switchback jogging left (north) away from Thunder Creek, near 18.1 mi (29.1 km), 4880 ft (1487 m), reach **Upper Thunder Basin camp**. Beyond, the trail ascends southeast. It then steepens, switchbacking generally east, before curving right (south) to crest **Park Creek Pass** at 19.8 mi (31.9 km), 6100 ft (1859 m).

Descending south-southeast from Park Creek Pass, the primary source of Park Creek is visible right (west): the glaciers on 9112-ft (2777-m) Buckner

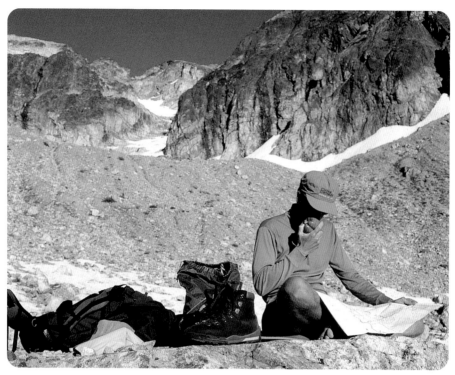

Park Creek Pass

Mtn. South of Buckner are the cliffs of 8280-ft (2524-m) Booker Mtn. Left (southeast) are 8515-ft (2595-m) Storm King Mtn and 9197-ft (2803-m) Goode Mtn. The trail plies heather meadows briefly before switchbacking down into Park Creek valley.

Reach **Buckner camp** at 22 mi (35.4 km) and pass Fivemile horse camp at 22.4 mi (36 km). Continue descending southeast into forest. Views are limited but for glimpses of Park Creek Ridge (southwest) and Goode Ridge (northeast).

At 25 mi (40.2 km) reach tiny **Twomile camp**. The trail departs upper Park Creek valley here, descending south then switchbacking southwest down to **Park Creek camp,** on upper Stehekin Valley Road, at 27 mi (43.5 km), 2300 ft (701 m).

Prior to the apocalyptic storm of 2003, the upper Stehekin Valley Road was indeed a road. In summer, buses shuttled hikers between Lake Chelan and Cottonwood camp. But the storm damage was so extensive the National Park Service permanently closed the upper 9.9 mi (15.9 km) of the 23-mi (37-km) road to vehicle traffic. Now a former road reverting to trail, it remains passable on foot. The Park Service intends to designate a new trail using parts of the old road between Bridge Creek and Cottonwood camp.

From Park Creek camp, left on the road/trail leads 3 mi (4.8 km) east to Bridge Creek. From there, the Pacific Crest Trail continues 12.8 mi (20.6 km) generally northeast to the Bridge Creek trailhead on Hwy 20, for a total one-way trip distance of 42.8 mi (68.9 km).

If proceeding from Park Creek camp to Cascade Pass, turn right on the road/trail and follow it 4 mi (6.4 km) generally northwest, upstream along the Stehekin River, to **Cottonwood camp** at 31 mi (50 km), 2800 ft (853 m).

On trail now, continue northwest along the verdant valley floor with views of forested slopes. Reach **Basin Creek camp** at 32.4 mi (52.1 km), 3160 ft (963 m). After a short, gradual ascent west, reach a junction at 33.4 mi (53.7 km), 3600 ft (1097 m).

Here, a right fork ascends 1.5 mi (2.5 km) east then north into Horseshoe Basin—an impressive cirque where cascades spill off Horseshoe Peak, Ripsaw Ridge, Boston Peak, and Sahale Mtn.

From the 33.4-mi (53.7-km) junction, follow the main trail left (west). Ascend a talus slope and at 34.1 mi (54.9 km), 4000 ft (1219 m), ford Doubtful Creek. The grade steepens beyond, switchbacking generally west, then traversing south.

The trail then curves northwest and the ascent eases. At 35.6 mi (57.3 km), 4800 ft (1463 m) reach **Pelton Basin camp** and the most appealing and scenic tentsites since Buckner camp. Here, wood tent platforms enable you to pitch your tent in open meadows without damaging them.

Resuming the gradual ascent northwest, continue probing Pelton Basin until cresting **Cascade Pass** at 36.4 mi (58.6 km), 5400 ft (1646 m). From here, a gently descending traverse north-northwest, then a switchbacking plunge west, lead to the end of the Cascade River Road. Enter the spacious trailhead parking lot at 40.1 mi (64.5 km), 3600 ft (1097 m).

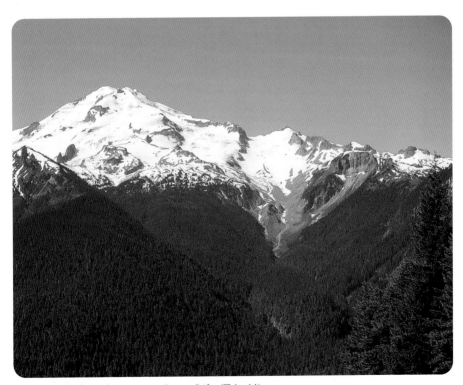

Glacier Peak, from the ascent to Image Lake (Trip 44).

IMAGE LAKE

LOCATION	Glacier Peak Wilderness
	Mt. Baker-Snoqualmie National Forest
ROUND TRIP	33.6 mi (54.1 km) to Image Lake
	44.6 mi (71.8 km) to Cloudy Pass
ELEVATION GAIN	4300 ft (1311 m) to Image Lake
	5238 ft (1597 m) to Cloudy Pass
KEY ELEVATIONS	trailhead 1800 ft (549 m), Image Lake 6056 ft (1846 m)
	Cloudy Pass 6438 ft (1962 m)
HIKING TIME	3 to 5 days
DIFFICULTY	challenging
MAPS	*Green Trails* Glacier Peak 112, Holden 113

OPINION

Once in a great while, you see an image that instantly earns a permanent place in your mental gallery, where you can return to it again and again for emotional renewal, perhaps even spiritual sustenance. The view of Glacier Peak from the aptly named Image Lake is such a sight.

Here, you're not staring up at the iconic mountain or gazing at it from afar. You're directly across from it, seemingly as high as the summit itself. Unless you're a climber with the skill to surmount Glacier Peak, Image Lake is the supreme vantage, the most auspicious site for a private audience with The Volcano God.

The trip begins with a long, meditative forest walk beside the Suiattle River. Tread is soft underfoot. The swift, powerful water is often within view the first few miles. Deep shade makes this a pleasant stretch even on a hot day. If it's not raining, all the mosses and ferns will remind you how lucky you are.

See the word *long* in the first sentence of the previous paragraph? Grok it. Upon returning to the trailhead, you'll have hiked below treeline for at least 27.6 mi (44.4 km). So be patient on your trek. Flow into it. The complex tapestry of this enchanted forest has the power to enthrall, if you'll let it. By expanding your awareness, rather than focusing on your agenda, perhaps when you finally emerge above treeline, you'll feel you've *grown* into the rapturous scenery rather than barged into it.

When you're ready for a change, the trail offers a radical one: a gravity-defying ordeal. The 4.7-mi (7.6-km), 3200-ft (975-m) climb to Miners Ridge is steep—an entirely new order of verticality, hence the third "e." You'll switchback at least two dozen times in just the lower 2.5-mi (4-km).

After 10 a.m. on a sunny, midsummer day, this slope can be hot enough to bake your enchilada. And there's no water beyond the first creek—a mere 0.75 mi (1.2 km) up. So it's wise to end day one by pitching your tent near the

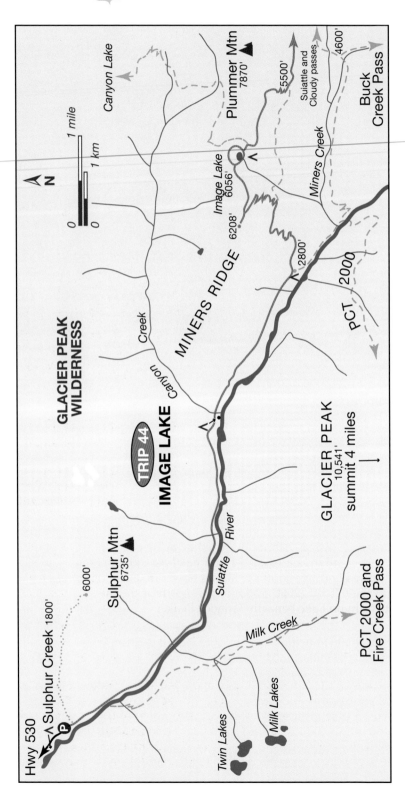

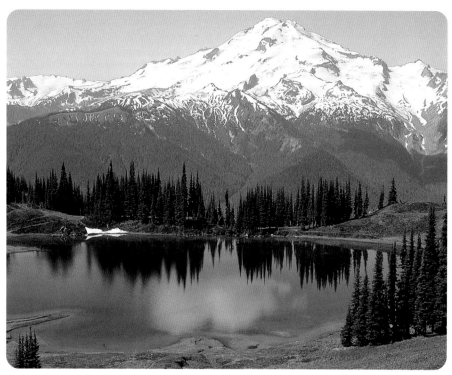

Image Lake and Glacier Peak

junction on the valley floor: 10.8 mi (17.4 km) from the trailhead. Then, on day two, fill your water bottles and start climbing by 7 a.m. It can take four or five hours to crest the ridge.

When the grade finally relents, Image Lake is still 1 km (1.6 mi) distant, but already you'll have been repaid: the panorama is empyrean. After pitching your tent in the basin southeast of the lake, break out your ultralight camp chair. Relax. Enjoy the rousing view of Glacier Peak. But not for long. Short, easy explorations beckon.

Definitely walk northeast up the heathery slope to the crest of Miners Ridge and wander east toward Plummer Mtn. You'll soon see a parade of jagged spires and overlook the alpine bowl surrounding Image Lake. Also walk up the 6758-ft (2060-m) knoll just north of the lake for a view farther north to Canyon Lake beneath Bannock Peak.

On day three, choose from two excursions. Canyon Lake is a 14.4-mi (23.1-km) round trip via a rough, unmaintained trail. In addition to the lake, you're sure to find solitude. But Cloudy Pass is the scenically superior option, plus it's closer: just 11 mi (17.7 km) round trip.

En route to Cloudy Pass, you'll follow the Miners Ridge trail—one of the North Cascades' all-time-great meadow walks. Just shy of Cloudy, you'll reach Suiattle Pass—a narrow, tree-choked notch of consequence only as a trail junction. Persist to Cloudy Pass, an alpine saddle on the shoulder of Cloudy Peak. The revelatory view here is a gratifying climax. Visible southeast are the Lyman Lakes, the Lyman Glacier, and the mountains bookending Spider Gap.

A choice of off-trail rambles lure strong hikers above Cloudy Pass for even better views. Head southwest 0.5 mi (0.8 km) to a knoll-top panorama that includes Glacier Peak (southwest). Or ascend higher yet, northeast toward Cloudy Peak.

Most people dayhike to Cloudy Pass from their Image Lake basecamp. On day four, they return to the trailhead via the Suiattle River trail. It's also possible, however, to move camp on day three to Cloudy Pass, then continue hiking a circuit back to the trailhead via Miners Creek.

If clear skies allowed you to fully appreciate the views at Image Lake and on Miners Ridge, descending via Miners Creek is worthwhile, adding another dimension to the journey. Also, the trail is forested, on a north-facing slope, so it provides foul-weather protection and afternoon shade, which the exposed Miners Ridge trail does not.

Whether you choose to make this a round trip (backpacking to Image Lake, then dayhiking to Cloudy Pass) or a circuit (backpacking to Image Lake, proceeding to Cloudy Pass, then continuing down Miners Creek), your total distance will be roughly the same. The round-trip plus dayhike, of course, spares you the burden of your full pack for a significant distance.

Dropping from Suiattle Pass on the Miners Creek trail, your legs will struggle to hold back your ready-to-roll body. The roar of the creek fills the valley here. The trail soon eases into a gradual descent through magnificent, ancient trees. We didn't see Sasquatch, but we're sure he lives here.

Upon reaching the Suiattle River, a right turn quickly leads to the junction where you previously began ascending to Image Lake. You're again on familiar ground. Simply follow the trail downstream to the trailhead.

BEFORE YOUR TRIP

Flood damage to Suiattle River Road 26 rendered the trailhead at Sulphur Creek campground inaccessible in 1991. The road was repaired and reopened to vehicle traffic, but the infamous 2003 storm washed it out again. The Forest Service, through a tedious grant process, eventually received funds to repair the road. The work began in 2006. Before the repairs were completed, however, the November '06 storm further damaged the road. Forest Service officials are optimistic the repair work will continue in 2007. For current conditions, contact the Darrington Ranger Station, or check recent trip reports submitted to the Washington Trails Association (www.wta.org). If the Suiattle River Road remains closed, consider hiking to Image Lake via Buck Creek Pass, or via Lake Chelan and Lyman Lake.

BY VEHICLE

Drive Hwy 530 south 11.3 mi (18.2 km) from Rockport, or north 7.2 mi (11.6 km) from Darrington. On the east side of the Sauk River bridge, turn east onto Suiattle River Road 26. Follow it 23 mi (37 km) southeast to Sulphur Creek campground. The road's end trailhead is just beyond, at 1800 ft (549 m).

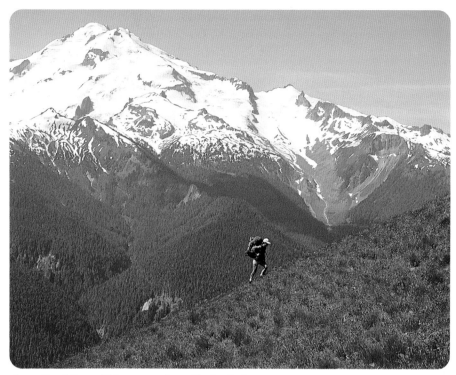

Ascending Miners Ridge, across from Glacier Peak

ON FOOT

The trail follows the Suiattle River upstream, southeast. Ignore the left fork climbing Sulphur Mtn's west face. At 0.8 mi (1.3 km) ignore the Milk Creek trail forking right to cross the river. Proceed straight, staying above the northeast bank.

At 6.5 mi (10.5 km), 2400 ft (732 m) cross **Canyon Creek**. There's a tentsite west of the creek, on the right. At 10.5 mi (16.9 km) reach more tentsites near another creek.

The trail forks at 10.8 mi (17.4 km), 2800 ft (853 m). For Image Lake, go left and begin ascending east. Right continues following the river upstream to a junction at 12.2 mi (19.6 km) with the Miners Creek trail from Suiattle Pass.

En route to Image Lake, cross a creek at 11.5 mi (18.5 km)—the last reliable water source until the lake. At 13.3 mi (21.4 km), 4800 ft (1463 m) fork left (north) where right leads directly east to Suiattle Pass.

Crest **Miners Ridge** and reach a junction at 15.5 mi (24.9 km), 6000 ft (1829 m). Drop your pack and walk 0.2 mi (0.3 km) left (northwest) along the ridge to the fire lookout. Dome Peak and Dome Glacier are visible north. Glacier Peak dominates the southern horizon.

After detouring to the lookout, follow the main trail east-southeast, curving northeast. The trail forks again at 16.3 mi (26.2 km), 6100 ft (1859 m), above **Image Lake**. Both forks circle the lake, which is at 6056 ft (1846 m). Right, around the south shore, leads 0.5 mi (0.8 km) to the campground in the basin southeast of the lake.

Though the lake is not visible from the campground, many tentsites have views of Glacier Peak. There's a creek nearby. To avoid attracting bears, but also as a precaution against marauding marmots, be sure to hang your food at night and whenever you leave your site.

To reach either Canyon Lake or Cloudy Pass, continue following the trail around the south shore of Image Lake. Fork right (southeast) where left circles the north shore. Reach a junction 0.2 mi (0.3 km) farther. Left (north) leads to Canyon Lake. Right is the Miners Ridge trail east to Cloudy Pass.

The rough, unmaintained trail to Canyon Lake ascends above Image Lake, descends east-southeast on the north side of Miners Ridge, then traverses north across the head of Canyon Creek basin. **Canyon Lake** is at 5700 ft (1737 m), beneath Bannock Peak. It's a 14.4-mi (23.2-km) round trip from Image Lake.

Cloudy Pass is an 11-mi (17.7-km) round trip from Image Lake. The Miners Ridge trail ascends briefly then contours east through flower-filled alpine meadows before descending 600 ft (183 km) to a junction at 5500 ft (1676 km). Right descends to the Suiattle River. Go left, again contouring east.

Pass tentsites near a stream cascading off Plummer Mtn just before reaching another junction at 5500 ft (1676 km). Proceed straight (east). Right (south) is the Miners Creek trail descending to the Suiattle River.

Soon pass a tentsite in a tiny meadow below the trail just before reaching a junction in forested **Suiattle Pass** at 5983 ft (1824 m). Left leads north past Sitting Bull Mtn. Bear right and continue northeast.

At the next junction, where left descends west into the South Fork Agnes Creek drainage, bear right again. A switchbacking ascent generally east tops out in 6438-ft (1962-m) **Cloudy Pass**. Distance from Image Lake: 5.5 mi (8.9 km). Elevation gain: 938 ft (286 m).

Bear in mind, the trail described here linking Suiattle and Cloudy passes is the short, direct route traversing a headwall and piercing a rough, rocky chute. After late July in a year of average snowfall, it should be snow-free and pose no problem. If icy, however, it could be precarious, in which case you can detour around it: return to Suiattle Pass, descend right (north), turn right (east) at the next two junctions, then go left (northeast) at the third.

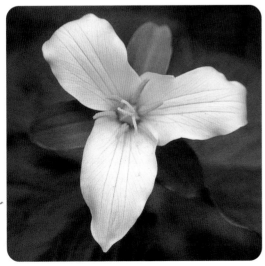

Trillium

At Cloudy Pass, you're surrounded by 7915-ft (2412-m) Cloudy Peak (northeast), 7759-ft (2365-m) Sitting Bull Mtn (northwest), 8674-ft (2644-m) Fortress Mtn (south), 8459-ft (2578-m) Chiwawa Mtn (south-southeast), and 8421-ft (2567-m) Dumbell Mtn southeast. Spider Gap is

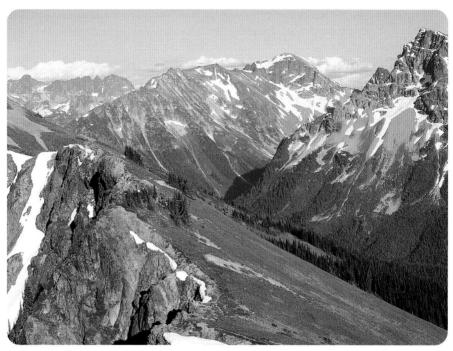

On Miners Ridge

between Chiwawa and Dumbell. The trail descends southeast to Lyman Lake, visible below, then continues to Holden, 10.4 mi (16.7 km) distant. From there, a road leads east 11 mi (17.7 km) to Lake Chelan.

If you're not dayhiking from Image Lake but are instead backpacking a circuit, upon returning to the first junction west of Suiattle Pass, turn left onto the Miners Creek trail. It descends south then west to cross **Miners Creek** at 4500 ft (1372 m).

After a gentle ascent south, reach a junction at 4600 ft (1402 m), 3.6 mi (5.8 km) from Suiattle Pass. Left leads south to Buck Creek Pass. Turn right and begin a long, gradual descent west through ancient forest.

At 2798 ft (852 m) reach a junction beside the **Suiattle River**, 8.4 mi (13.5 km) from Suiattle Pass. Left crosses the river to traverse Glacier Peak's north slope. Turn right and follow the river downstream (northwest) along the northeast bank. There are tentsites here, among tall trees.

Quickly reach **Miners Creek**, which you must ford if no log crossing is available. Shortly beyond—9.8 mi (15.8 km) from Suiattle Pass—reach the junction where you initially ascended to Image Lake. You're now on familiar ground. Bear left and follow the Suiattle River trail 10.8 mi (17.4 km) downstream, generally northwest, back to the **Suiattle River trailhead**, where your total circuit distance will be 45 mi (72.4 km).

LOST CREEK RIDGE / LAKE BYRNE

LOCATION	Glacier Peak Wilderness
ROUND TRIP	21.4 mi (34.4 km)
ELEVATION GAIN	5060 ft (1542 m)
KEY ELEVATIONS	trailhead 1900 ft (580 m), highpoint 5923 ft (1806 m) Lake Byrne 5800 ft (1768 m)
HIKING TIME	2 days
DIFFICULTY	moderate
MAPS	*Green Trails* Sloan Peak 111, Glacier Peak 112

OPINION

Our planet loses more than an acre (0.4 hectare) of wilderness every 15 seconds. It's devoured by logging, housing construction, road building, and commercial development.

In the North Cascades, violent storms—that in expert opinion are caused by global warming—have ravaged roads and trails, making it difficult or impossible for hikers to access what little wilderness remains.

Cherish the few untouched enclaves. Appreciate the existing byways and footpaths. Drive your Toyota Prius (bearing a "Daddy, what were trees like?" bumper sticker) out of the city, then follow this rough, ridge-riding trail into the raw, back-of-beyond, where you'll see one of the world's most majestic sights: Glacier Peak, from Lake Byrne.

Afterward, you'll be more inspired than ever to vote for environmentally-minded representatives, to donate to groups like the Washington Trails Association, and to keep exploring the North Cascades.

This perspective of the icy volcano's western slope reveals a crater more jagged than Mt. Baker's. You'll also see the Kennedy and Scimitar glaciers clawing at the peak from sky to forest. But the Lost Creek Ridge trail isn't a one-view wonder. You'll see the surrounding summits and valleys en route.

In '03 and '06, calamitous storms devastated the White Chuck River trail, destroyed Kennedy Hot Springs, and ruined portions of the Pacific Crest Trail beyond. As a result, the only reasonable access to Lake Byrne is now via Lost Creek Ridge.

That's not to say the ridge route is inferior to the previous options, but that—for all except the hardiest bush-bashing baboons—Lake Byrne is now the destination of a one way, in-and-out backpack trip, rather than the scenic climax of a longer loop.

For most of us, the ridge itself poses enough challenge. It's steep. The trail is often narrow, eroded, faint. In places, the tread is only as wide as your boot is long. Where it traverses precipitous slopes, you must step carefully, with full awareness, especially if you're forced by time constraints to hike during rain or at dusk.

THE REI GUARANTEE

Our 100% guarantee
ensures that every item you
purchase at REI meets your
high standards—or you can return
it for a replacement or refund

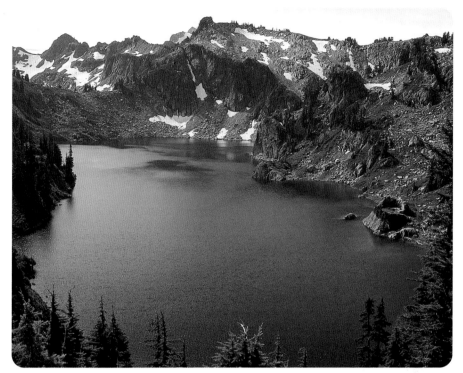

Lake Byrne atop Lost Creek Ridge

Your compensation will be a sense of adventure that tamer, more populous trails don't offer. That's especially true when you're surfing the 6.2-mi (10-km) crest of Lost Creek Ridge and exploring the panoramic vantage points above Lake Byrne.

If you don't get that early start you were hoping for, and you're unable to reach the Camp Lake tentsites just shy of Lake Byrne, don't worry. After passing Round Lake Junction, you'll find inviting places to bed down along the ridge.

BY VEHICLE

From the east side of Granite Falls, drive the Mountain Loop Hwy east 30.75 mi (49.5 km) to Barlow Pass. Curve left (north) and continue 7.2 mi (11.6 km). Or, from Darrington, drive the Mountain Loop Hwy southeast 16.5 mi (10.2 km). From either approach, turn southeast onto North Fork Sauk River Road 49. Follow it 3.1 mi (5 km) to the Lost Creek Ridge trailhead, on the left, at 1900 ft (580 m).

ON FOOT

Heading generally northeast, the trail crosses a creek plummeting off Spring Mtn (left / north). Soon begin a steep, switchbacking ascent through forest.

Near 2700 ft (823 m) the trail curves north, still switchbacking. Reach 4360-ft (1330-m) **Bingley Gap** at 3.3 mi (5.3 km). Here the trail veers right (east), ascending the crest of Lost Creek Ridge.

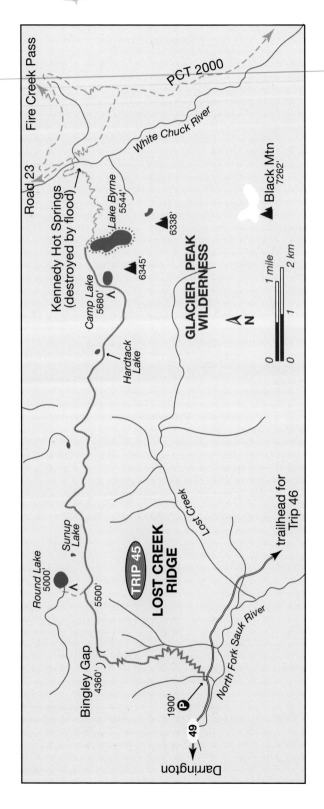

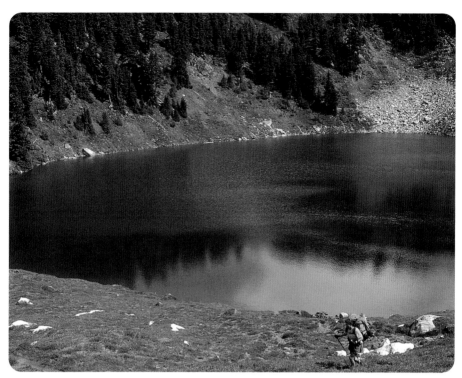

Camp Lake

Reach a junction at 4.6 mi (7.4 km), 5500 ft (1677 m). Left descends north to tentsites at **Round Lake**, visible 500 ft (152 m) below and 0.7 mi (1.1 km) distant. The main trail proceeds generally east, soon passing above Sunup Lake (left / north). You've gained 3600 ft (1098 m) so far.

Just beyond Round Lake junction are passable tentsites. You'll also find streams trickling through a rocky basin. In moist, grassy areas here, look for a rare wildflower: the waxy, deep purple, king gentian.

Though eroded and narrow, the trail remains evident—among trees, across rock, through heather—on a series of ups and downs. At 7 mi (11.3 km), it shifts to the south side of the ridgecrest, granting a view of Black and Red mountains (southeast and south-southeast), Sloan Peak (southwest), and the North Fork Sauk River canyon (southwest).

Pass reasonable tentsites near 7.5 mi (12 km). Meadow Mtn is visible north at 8 mi (12.9 km). So far you've hiked about 5 mi (8 km) along the ridge, gaining and losing approximately 300 ft (91 m) in the process. Ahead the trail climbs another 300 ft (91 m) to the 5923-ft (1806-m) **highpoint**, then descends. Attain a view east to Glacier Peak. Pass Hardtack Lake (a mere pond) at 8.5 mi (13.7 km), 5700 ft (1738 m).

Proceed southeast, then curve north to reach **Camp Lake** at 10 mi (16.1 km), 5680 ft (1732 m). Surrounded by gentle, meadowy slopes, it offers a couple good tentsites. Camp here, because the tiny meadows around Lake Byrne are less accommodating and more fragile.

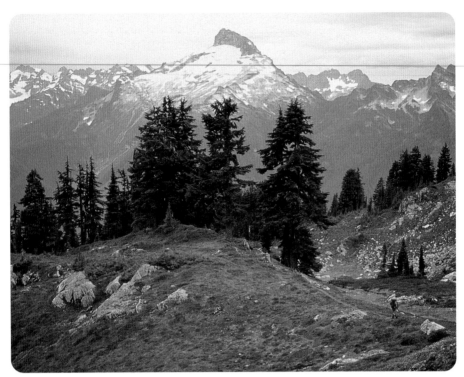

Sloan Peak, from Lost Creek Ridge near Round Lake junction

Continuing northeast, the Lake Byrne cirque is visible 250 ft (76 m) below. The trail skirts the north end of **Lake Byrne** at 10.7 mi (17.2 km), 5800 ft (1768 m). The lake is at 5544 ft (1690 m).

It's possible to scramble around the lake on the ridges above. The optimal viewpoints are the 6338-ft (1932-m) knoll south of Lake Byrne, and the 6345-ft (1934-m) ridge between Lake Byrne and Camp Lake. Directly south of Lake Byrne is 7262-ft (2214-m) Black Mtn.

Make this an out-and-back trip, returning to the trailhead via Lost Creek Ridge. The rough trail does continue, however, east then northeast, plunging 2300 ft (700 m) in 2.5 mi (4 km) to intersect the White Chuck River trail. But the ensuing loop options are now fraught with difficulty.

This drainage was severely damaged by the '03 and '06 storms. Kennedy Hot Springs used to be here. It's now gone, buried beneath flood debris. Long stretches of the trail following the White Chuck River downstream (northwest) 5.2 mi (8.1 km) to the White Chuck trailhead were washed away. Where the trail remains, toppled trees are a constant obstacle.

On the Pacific Crest Trail, which follows the river upstream (south) to Red Pass, bridges previously spanning Sitkum Creek, Baekos Creek, and the upper White Chuck were swept away. Long sections of the trail are now obscure.

Repairing the damage requires more money than is currently available and could take years. For current conditions, contact the Darrington Ranger Station, or check recent trip reports submitted to the Washington Trails Association (www.wta.org).

PILOT RIDGE / WHITE PASS

LOCATION	Glacier Peak Wilderness
CIRCUIT	29.1 mi (46.8 km)
ELEVATION GAIN	6000 ft (1830 m)
KEY ELEVATIONS	trailhead 2100 ft (640 m), Pilot Ridge 6160 ft (1878 m)
	Blue Lake 5625 ft (1715 m)
	shortcut highpoint 6360 ft (1940 m)
	Dishpan Gap 5600 ft (1707 m)
	Indian Pass 5000 ft (1524 m), White Pass 5904 ft (1800 m)
	Mackinaw shelter 3000 ft (915 m)
HIKING TIME	3 days
DIFFICULTY	challenging
MAPS	*Green Trails* Sloan Peak 111, Glacier Peak 112
	Benchmark Mtn 144

OPINION

St. Peter's is not Rome. Disney World is not Florida. Glacier Peak is not Glacier Peak Wilderness. Landmarks often deceive. Overshadowed by a dominating mountain, the scenery in this immense wilderness is more marvelously varied than you might think. That's why this is a premier backpack trip. Your enjoyment won't depend on seeing Glacier Peak. It's only one of many powerful sights.

You'll witness the first within minutes of leaving the trailhead: ancient, giant trees. Saved from the saw, the North Fork Sauk River valley harbors firs and cedars so big, so numerous, it inspires comparison with Olympic National Park's Hoh Rain Forest, and Mt. Rainier National Park's Grove of the Patriarchs. And on this journey, you'll walk the entire North Fork valley. Some people come here to do nothing but. Rather than wait until summer to backpack the circuit, they come in spring or fall simply to dayhike the valley bottom as far as Red Creek. Keep it in mind as a shoulder-season option.

The next arresting sight on this trip comes after you've endured the steep ascent to the crest of Pilot Ridge. Here you'll see the tremendous Monte Cristo massif. No other hiker-accessible vantage reveals its full stature like this one does. Glacier Peak soon leaps into view as well, of course, but so do many other notable mountains, including Sloan Peak, Pugh Mtn, Mt. Baker, even Mt. Rainier.

The ascent from the North Fork valley to Pilot Ridge is the only leg of the journey that's all work and no wow. Once you're atop the crest, the work gradually diminishes and the wows resume, their frequency and magnitude gradually increasing. Pilot, however, is like most ridges: decidedly unlevel. Walking it, you feel like a tiny ship in rough seas, cresting waves then plunging into troughs. But the meadows you'll eventually traverse are so long and languorous they more than compensate.

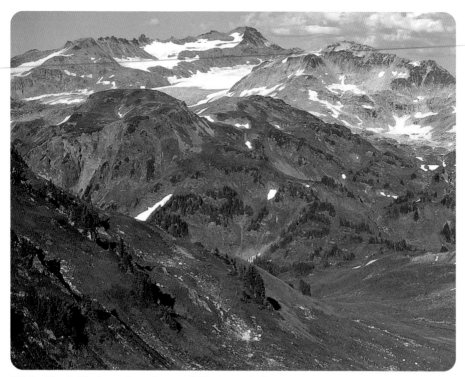

White Chuck Glacier and south arm of Glacier Peak, from Red Pass

If you simply stay on the trail, following our directions, you're assured of a highly scenic experience. But three deviations are so spectacular, you shouldn't think of them as optional: White Mtn, Red Pass, and Portal Peak. None is long or difficult. Each is described below. Red Pass is especially easy. Include all in your plans.

Which way should you hike the circuit? It's a coin toss. Both directions have pros and cons. We describe it counter-clockwise, starting with the ascent of Pilot Ridge. That way, if it's hot, your steepest climb will be through forest, probably in the cool of the morning; rather than on a sun-pummeled slope in the afternoon.

Because there's no desirable campsite and little water on Pilot Ridge, start early and hike all the way to Blue Lake the first day. It's a rigorous 11.7 mi (18.8 km), but doable if you're strong.

From Pilot Ridge until you descend back into the North Fork valley, you'll be mostly in the subalpine zone where there are few trees for shade or shelter. Your protection from sun or inclement weather will be what you're wearing or carrying. If it's wet, you'll get very wet; if it's hot, you'll be very hot. Clear skies are almost a necessity for enjoying high-elevation trails like this, but when the temperature soars you'll want a wide-brimmed hat and maybe a bandana you can moisten and wrap around your neck. Fill your water bottles at every opportunity. Except in the North Fork valley, the trail can be dry for long stretches.

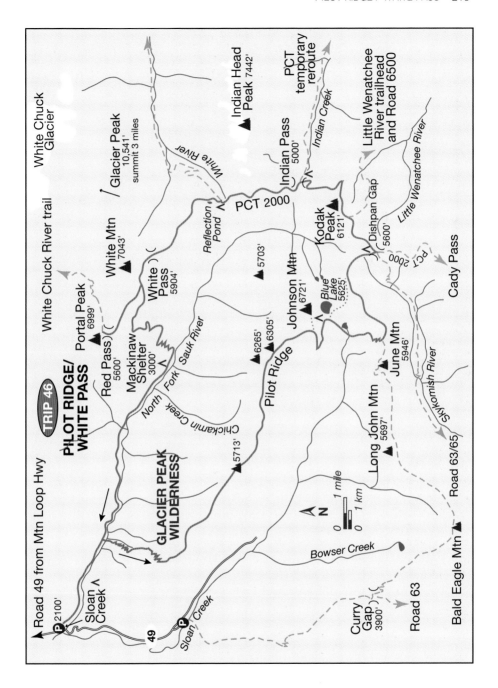

Road 49 from Mtn Loop Hwy

White Chuck Glacier

White Chuck River trail

TRIP 46

PILOT RIDGE/ WHITE PASS

Glacier Peak
10,541'
summit 3 miles

Indian Head
Peak 7442'

PCT temporary reroute

Little Wenatchee
River trailhead
and Road 6500

White Mtn
7043'

White River

Indian Pass
5000'

Indian Creek

Little Wenatchee River

Portal Peak
6999'

Reflection
Pond

PCT 2000

White
Pass
5904'

Kodak
Peak
6121'

Dishpan Gap
5600'

Cady Pass

Red Pass)
5600'

Mackinaw
Shelter
3000'

5703'

Johnson Mtn
6721'

Blue
Lake
5625'

PCT 2000

North Fork   Sauk River

6265'
6305'

Pilot Ridge

Chickamin Creek

5713'

June Mtn
5946'

Skykomish River

**GLACIER PEAK
WILDERNESS**

Long John Mtn
5697'

Road 63/65

N

0   1 mile
0   1 km

Bowser Creek

Sloan
Creek

49

Sloan Creek

Curry
Gap
3900'

Road 63

Bald Eagle Mtn

P 2100'

P

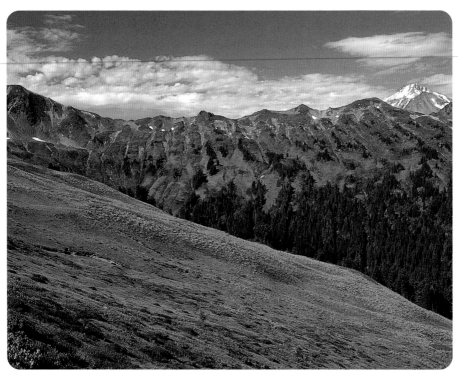

Looking north from lower White Pass

FACT

BY VEHICLE

From the east side of Granite Falls, drive the Mountain Loop Hwy east 30.75 mi (49.5 km) to Barlow Pass, then continue northeast 7.2 mi (11.6 km). Or, from Darrington, drive the Mountain Loop Hwy southeast 16.5 mi (26.6 km) toward Barlow Pass. (Pavement ends at 9.5 mi / 15.3 km).

From either approach, turn east onto North Fork Sauk River Road 49. At 6.7 mi (10.8 km) fork left. Reach the trailhead parking area at 6.8 mi (10.9 km), 2100 ft (640 m). The road ends just beyond, at Sloan Creek campground.

ON FOOT

Begin hiking southeast into ancient forest. A few minutes along, ignore the Red Mtn spur forking left (north). The trail is soon near the North Fork Sauk River, following it upstream.

At 1.9 mi (3.1 km), 2400 ft (732 m) reach a junction. The North Fork trail continues straight, upstream, to White Pass. That will be your return route. To hike the counter-clockwise circuit described below, turn right (south) and find a logjam on which to cross the river.

On the south bank, the trail begins a steep, switchbacking climb generally south-southwest, assaulting the northwest end of Pilot Ridge.

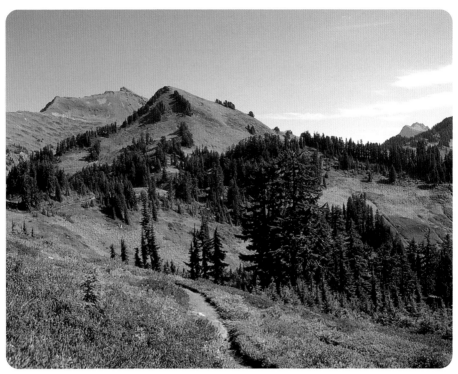

On the PCT, heading from Dishpan Gap to Kodak Peak

Cross a creeklet at about 3.8 mi (6.1 km), 4000 ft (1219 m). This is the last dependable water on the the entire ridge, so tank up. Shortly beyond, at 4.3 mi (6.9 km), is the first possible tentsite: a small level spot beside the trail.

At 4.6 mi (7.4 km) a rockslide splits the forest, which is mostly big, healthy hemlocks. At 5.1 mi (8.2 km), cross an unreliable creeklet. Glacier Peak is now visible northeast. Soon after, Red Mtn is visible north. Reach the narrow, northwest end of **Pilot Ridge** at 5.4 mi (8.7 km), 5400 ft (1646 m).

The steep ascent continues and the view improves. Visible northeast, from left to right, are Black Mtn, Portal Peak above Red Pass, and White Mtn above White Pass.

The panorama soon expands to include Mt. Baker and Pugh Mtn (northwest), the massive glacier on Sloan Peak (nearby west), the Monte Cristo massif (southwest), Mt. Rainier (distant south), the Alpine Lakes Wilderness (southeast), and the Icicle Group (east). Below (southwest) are the Sloan and Cadet creek valleys, at the base of Monte Cristo Peak.

Enter heather and berry bushes atop the ridge. Heading southeast, the trail is in the open for 0.3 mi (0.5 km), then in forest. It's level for about 0.5 mi (0.8 km), plunges 240 ft (73 m), then levels again in forest.

At 6.9 mi (11.1 km) the trail crosses a flat spot where you could, if necessary, pitch a tent. Finally, the ridgecrest is mostly level for 1 mi (0.6 km). At 8.5 mi (13.7 km)—on the right, in trees, just below the trail—is another adequate tentsite.

The walking is easier where the trail contours southeast across subalpine slopes. At 10.4 mi (16.7 km), 6160 ft (1878 m), go right (west) where a left (east) spur ascends Johnson Mtn. If you peer over the slope, Little Blue Lake is visible south.

At 11.4 mi (18.3 km), 5500 ft (1676 m), reach a **junction**. Left is the scenic-but-steep shortcut skirting Blue Lake's south shore. Right is the main trail southwest past Little Blue Lake to a junction near June Mtn, where left leads northeast to rejoin the shortcut.

Opting for the shortcut, go left (southeast). Ascend past a tentsite on the left, above the lake. Reach **Blue Lake** at 11.7 mi (18.8 km), 5625 ft (1715 m), in a steep-sided grassy bowl that restricts camping to only a few sites.

The shortcut trail ascends steeply from the lake's south shore. Heading generally south-southeast, it soon tops out in a 6360-ft (1940-m) **cleft** between knolls. There's just enough room here for a small tent. The view is extensive: northeast to Indian Head Peak, south to Mounts Daniels and Hinman, The Cradle in Alpine Lakes Wilderness, even Mt. Rainier.

From the gap, the trail leads east, abruptly descending a steep, rocky buttress, intersecting the main trail (from Little Blue Lake and June Mtn) at 12.5 mi (20.1 km), 5800 ft (1768 m). Go left (southeast, curving south) through meadows to a junction with the PCT in **Dishpan Gap** at 13.3 mi (21.4 km), 5600 ft (1707 m).

The gap is a broad, flat meadow, dotted with tarns, rimmed by hemlocks. There are campsites here, but it's a busy crossroads, so don't expect solitude. Right descends east to follow the Skykomish River downstream. Ahead, the PCT leads south, eventually to Hwy 2 near Stevens Pass. Go left, following the PCT generally northeast through subalpine meadows.

At 14 mi (22.5 km) and 14.2 mi (22.9 km) ignore trails dropping right (southeast) into Meander Meadow, unless you want to camp in the basin.

At 14.9 mi (24 km), 5600 ft (1707 m) ignore the Wenatchee Ridge trail forking right (east). Here the PCT turns sharply north, offering an unobstructed view northeast to 7442-ft (2268-m) Indian Head Peak. You've now rounded the base of **Kodak Peak**. If you need water, look for trailside seeps near 15.4 mi (24.8 km), on Kodak's northeast slope.

Descend north to reach 5000-ft (1524-m) **Indian Pass** at 15.9 mi (25.6 km). The pass is forested and has sheltered campsites. Small meadows and brackish tarns are surrounded by hemlocks. Ignore the Indian Creek trail (now the PCT detour) forking right and descending east-southeast. Proceed northwest, then generally north.

At 17.9 mi (28.8 km), 5400 ft (1646 m) ignore the White River trail forking right and descending northeast. There are campsites here. You'll find more campsites a bit farther, among the trees near Reflection Pond, at 18.2 mi (29.3 km).

Enter **White Pass** at 20.2 mi (32.5 km), 5904 ft (1800 m). Above you, straight ahead (north), is 7043-ft (2147-m) White Mtn. A 0.6-mi (1-km), cross-country ascent will grant you the summit and a commanding view: up at the White Chuck Glacier on Glacier Peak, down into the headwaters valley of the White Chuck River. Camping is prohibited at White Pass but allowed in the basin immediately below, accessed via the left (west) spur.

About 30 yd/m beyond, ignore a right (east) spur descending into Foam Basin. Proceed straight (north). At 20.6 mi (33.2 km) reach a water source: several rivulets pouring off White Mtn.

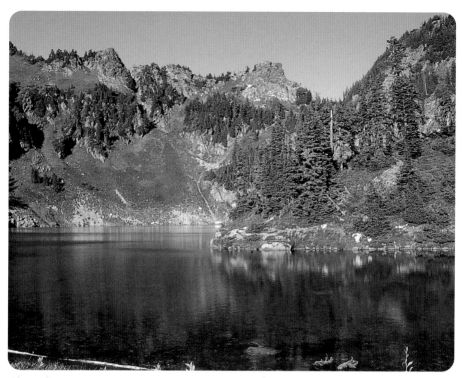

Blue Lake

The trail forks at 20.9 mi (33.6 km), 6000 ft (1830 m). Right leads northwest 1.7 mi (2.7 km) to 6500-ft (1981-m) **Red Pass** below Portal Peak, then descends east into the headwater drainage of the White Chuck River, where the historic '03 storm destroyed the PCT and necessitated the Indian Creek detour.

Proceeding to Red Pass, however, is easy and scenically rewarding. Ascending to the 6999-ft (2133-m) summit of Portal Peak will broaden your panorama. Competent scramblers can continue north-northwest from Portal Peak, over Skullcap Peak, to Black Mtn, then west to Red Mtn. From there, if you're skilled and determined, it's even possible to descend past Ruby Lake to Road 49, near the North Fork Sauk River trailhead.

To complete your circuit via the North Fork Sauk River valley trail, go left at the 20.9-mi (33.6-km) junction and descend initially east. You'll drop 3000 ft (915 km) en route to the valley floor. Reach **Mackinaw shelter**, a ramshackle lean-to near the river, at 23.7 mi (38.1 km), 3000 ft (915 m). There are several tentsites here.

Follow the trail downstream (northwest), along the north bank, through deep, cool, virgin forest. Find a log on which to cross Red Creek, or de-boot and ford it. At 27.2 mi (43.8 km) pass the left (south) fork where you previously crossed the river to ascend Pilot Ridge. You're now on familiar ground. Proceed straight, generally northwest, above the north bank. Reach the **trailhead** parking area at 29.1 mi (46.8 km), 2100 ft (640 m).

TRIP 47
BUCK CREEK PASS

LOCATION	Glacier Peak Wilderness / Wenatchee National Forest
ROUND TRIP	19.2 mi (31 km)
ELEVATION GAIN	3100 ft (945 m)
KEY ELEVATIONS	trailhead 2800 ft (853 m), pass 5900 ft (1798 m)
HIKING TIME	2 days
DIFFICULTY	moderate
MAP	*Green Trails* Holden 113

OPINION

Idyllic meadows undulate from pass to pass. Glacier Peak crowds out the sky. Ice-laden Clark Mtn vies for attention with the great volcano. High Pass, above Triad Lake, bears comparison with Sahale Arm or the Enchantment Lakes. The deep, green Suiattle River valley adds dimension to the scene.

All this and more awaits those who endure the dusty, cheerless trail to Buck Creek Pass.

And it *will* test your endurance. The heat is often enervating here. The disenchanted forest fails to inspire. The bugs will badger you. The sustained lack of scenery is disheartening.

But exultation will kick in about a mile below your destination. Upon cresting Buck Creek Pass, you can choose from several compelling explorations.

Traipsing south into the nearby alplands is a must. In season, profuse lupine and paintbrush carpet the meadowy slopes of Liberty Cap. (See inside back cover for a view northeast from Liberty Cap.) Continue farther south— past icy Triad Lake, toward massive, angular Buck Mtn—to High Pass, where you can stare into the green depths of remote Napeequa River valley.

Another easy goal is the pastoral summit of Flower Dome, a mere 1 mi (1.6 km) west-northwest of Buck Creek Pass. Yet another is the basin east of Helmet Butte, south of Pass No Pass. From here, scramblers can summit the 7366-ft (2245-m) butte or even 8674-ft (2644-m) Fortress Mtn.

Now, back down to earth for a moment. In more than 1500 mi (2415 km) of trekking through the North Cascades, our worst experience with black flies was here. Expect a satanic scourge until you escape up the Buck Creek valley headwall. In midsummer, 60 of them will be crawling on you the minute you stand still.

What to do? They don't show up for work until it gets warm, around 10 a.m., so start hiking before 7 a.m. Be prepared to eschew rest stops for the first 8 mi (12.9 km). Slurping water and chuffing down snacks on the go will prevent them from swarming you. They usually go to bed as soon as it cools off, around 5 p.m., so begin your return hike from Buck Creek Pass after

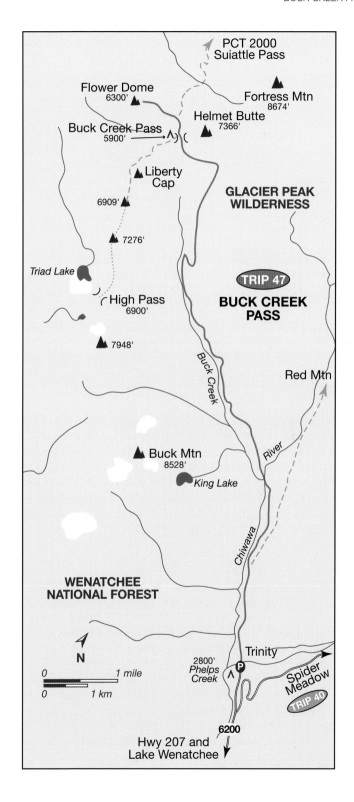

PCT 2000
Suiattle Pass

Flower Dome
6300'

Fortress Mtn
8674'

Helmet Butte
7366'

Buck Creek Pass
5900'

Liberty
Cap

6909'

GLACIER PEAK
WILDERNESS

7276'

Triad Lake

TRIP 47

BUCK CREEK
PASS

High Pass
6900'

7948'

Buck Creek

Red Mtn

River

Buck Mtn
8528'

King Lake

Chiwawa

WENATCHEE
NATIONAL FOREST

N

0   1 mile
0   1 km

Trinity

2800'
Phelps
Creek

P

Spider
Meadow

TRIP 40

6200

Hwy 207 and
Lake Wenatchee

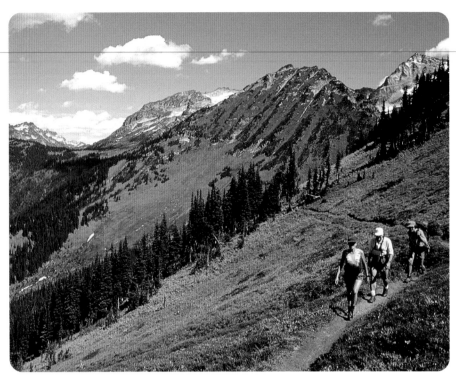

Heading to Liberty Cap, from Buck Creek Pass

3 p.m. Try bringing a bevy of friends with you. Together you'll stay sane by keeping the mood light and distracting each other from your misery.

Robo-hikers can smoke the trail to Buck Creek Pass on a Saturday, then visit High Pass and hike all the way out on Sunday. But most people should allow at least three days, devoting the second day to high-elevation discovery.

FACT

BY VEHICLE

Drive Hwy 2 to Coles Corner, 19.5 mi (31.4 km) east of Stevens Pass, or 16 mi (25.7 km) northwest of Leavenworth. Turn north onto Hwy 207, reset your trip odometer to zero, and proceed toward Lake Wenatchee. Pass the state park and the road to Plain. At 4.3 mi (6.9 km), go right (east) toward the Chiwawa Loop Road. At 5.7 mi (9.2 km) turn left onto Meadow Creek Road, which leads north to Fish Lake and the Chiwawa River valley. Pavement ends at 16.8 mi (27 km). Fork left at 28.1 mi (45.2 km). Pass Phelps Creek campground on the left at 28.4 mi (45.7 km). Reach the trailhead parking lot at 28.7 mi (46.2 km), 2800 ft (853 m).

ON FOOT

Cross the bridge to the northwest bank of Phelps Creek. The trail initially meanders around the Trinity mining operation.

Bear left at 0.4 mi (0.7 km). You're now on an old road. At the next fork, go

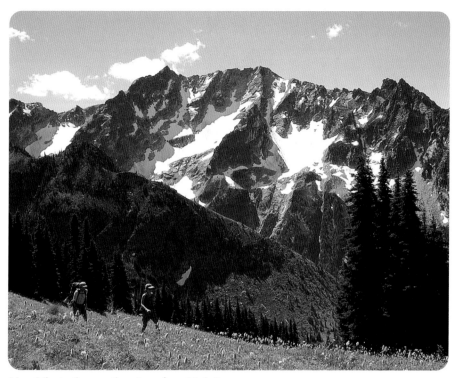

Near Liberty Cap, on the return from High Pass

right. Enter Glacier Peak Wilderness at 0.7 mi (1.1 km). The road soon dwindles to trail.

Reach a junction at 1.4 mi (2.3 km), 3100 ft (945 m). Right leads north to Red Mtn. Go left and proceed north-northwest. The forest is more verdant after 1.7 mi (2.7 km).

Cross the **Chiwawa River** bridge at 3 mi (4.8 km). There are campsites above the west bank. So far, the elevation gain has been negligible. Begin a moderate ascent through drier forest.

Near 4 mi (6.4 km), just before a meadow, Buck Mtn is visible left (southwest). Its 8528-ft (2600-m) summit is 5000 ft (1524 m) above you. Here the ascent northwest begins in earnest, but long switchbacks allow a comfortable pace.

Pass a stream and a level campsite at 5.7 mi (9.2 km). Proceed through tall, dense timber. Pass a larger campsite at 6 mi (10 km). The valley narrows and both walls are now visible. Rocky escarpments and green avalanche slopes distinguish the southwest wall.

At 7 mi (11.3 km) cross a huge **avalanche swath**. Though the snowslide occurred in the mid 90s, it's still evident where it shredded the opposite valley wall, then careened up the northeast wall where you are.

On a switchback at 7.5 mi (12 km) the trail veers sharply right, away from Buck Creek, then begins ascending steeply northwest. Gain 600 ft (183 m) in the next 0.8 mi (1.3 km). The grade then eases on a high traverse.

Near 8.3 mi (13.4 km) the forest opens, revealing the headwaters of Buck Creek, the forested pass, and the meadowy slopes of **Helmet Butte**. Water is available at 8.8 mi (14.2 km), where a right spur ascends north into the basin below Pass No Pass.

At 9.6 mi (15.4 km), 5900 ft (1798 m), reach a slope just above **Buck Creek Pass**. There's a creeklet at the south end of the pass. Campsites are scattered among the trees below the southeast side. Trail 789 continues northwest to Middle Ridge, reaching Suiattle Pass at 18 mi (29 km).

To reach High Pass, take the trail dropping into Buck Creek Pass. Follow it south through trees and meadows 0.25 mi (0.4 km) and pick up signed trail 1562.2. It jogs right (northwest), around the ridge. Once on the ridge, it turns south. There's no reliable water source beyond, so carry plenty.

The trail ascends through grass and heather on the west side of Liberty Cap. Miners Ridge and Plummer Mtn, above the Suiattle River valley, are visible north. Dome Peak is beyond. Glacier-shouldered, 8602-ft (2622-m) Clark Mtn is south.

About 1.75 mi (2.8 km) from Buck Creek Pass, enter an open saddle at 6400 ft (1950 m). To the west, Glacier Peak looms large. North-northeast, beyond Helmet Butte, is Fortress Mtn. The trail you hiked to the pass is visible below (east) in Buck Creek valley.

Continue following the narrow, increasingly rough, sometimes very steep path generally south along the ridgecrest. A 7276-ft (2218-m) bump affords such a grand view that you might be inclined to end the excursion here. Triad Lake is visible directly south.

The path, however, does proceed to 7000-ft (2134-m) **High Pass**—about 4 mi (6.4 km) from Buck Creek Pass, above and slightly beyond Triad Lake. The new panorama here includes the lonely Napeequa River valley (south) and an even closer view of Clark Mtn beyond.

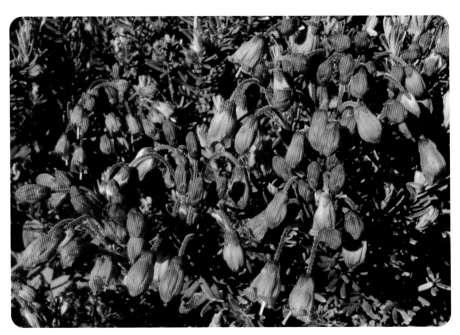

Heather

TRIP 48
PYRAMID MOUNTAIN

LOCATION	Chelan Mountains / Wenatchee National Forest
ROUND TRIP	18.4 mi (29.6 km)
ELEVATION GAIN	2800 ft (853 m) to, plus 1100 ft (335 m) from
KEY ELEVATIONS	trailhead 6500 ft (1981 m), summit 8245 ft (2513 m)
HIKING TIME	10 hours or 2 days
DIFFICULTY	challenging dayhike, easy backpack
MAP	*Green Trails* Lucerne 114

OPINION

North America's deepest gorge is not the Grand Canyon in Arizona. It isn't Hell's Canyon, on the Oregon-Idaho border. Nor is it Mexico's Copper Canyon.

It's Chelan Gorge, on the east edge of the North Cascades, where the mountains abruptly rise more than 8000 ft (2438 m) from the 1100-ft (335-m) shore of Lake Chelan.

Not only is this the deepest gorge, it actually *looks* like a gorge. Its walls average less than 2 mi (3.2 km) apart.

At its deepest, Chelan Gorge is 386 ft (118 m) below sea level. And that low-point is a short distance due east of your destination on this hike: Pyramid Mtn.

The long, sinuous lake is 7145 ft (2178 m) directly below the summit. But being a former fire-lookout site, Pyramid has a view of more than just water. The alps of Glacier Peak Wilderness are northwest, and those of Lake Chelan-Sawtooth Wilderness are east across the lake. Though no particular mountain or ridge dominates the horizon, the enormity of the spectacle is dazzling. And in all that vastness, there's virtually nothing of human construction in sight.

Pyramid is a long way from anywhere most people would consider anyplace at all. Hikers from Puget Sound are disinclined to drive clear across the range. And the nearest towns are tiny ones where excitement-starved youths favor dirt bikes over backpacks. That means you might well have the mountain to yourself.

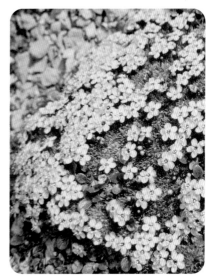

Moss campion

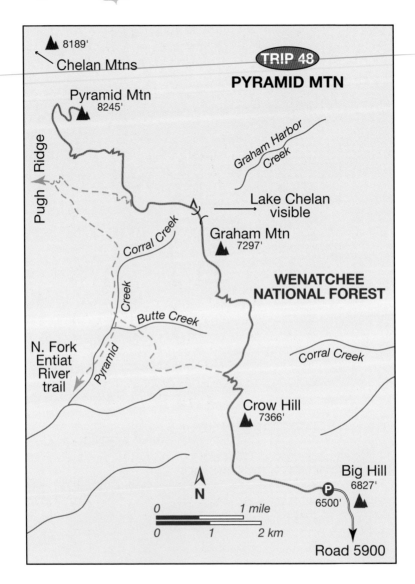

Fortunately, those obnoxiously loud motorcycles are prohibited on this trail. So in addition to solitude, you'll likely enjoy silence here. The terrain is arid, too, so there aren't even any water sounds to interrupt the tranquility. The buzz of an insect, maybe. A zephyr rustling the larch needles, perhaps. But that's it. Plus, at this altitude, there are fewer trees and more sky. The resulting spaciousness somehow amplifies the silence, making it more profound.

The Pyramid Mtn environs are high and dry. The trail is sometimes gravel, often dusty. Grass grows in tussocks instead of carpet-like meadows. The forests are open, the trees unimpressive. The sky is frequently brilliant blue. And the billowing, white cumulus clouds usually dissipate before turning mean. Pack plenty of water and fill up at every opportunity.

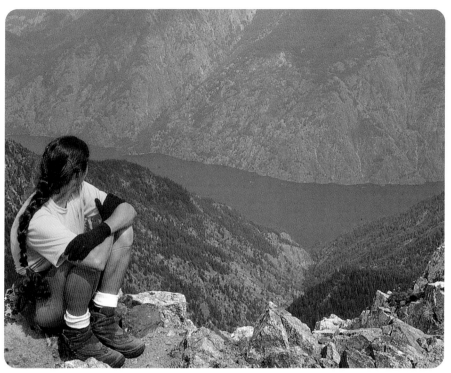

On summit of Pyramid Mountain—7145 ft (2178 m) above Lake Chelan

Looking at a map, you'll see it's possible to make Pyramid a circuit hike. Don't, unless you want to plod through boring forest. Return the same way, on the high route, and savor the views again.

Dayhiking Pyramid via the route described here takes about ten hours, but is enjoyable if you're up to the challenge. Afterward you can car camp at the trailhead or the Shady Pass Road junction. At either place you'll still probably be alone.

FACT

BY VEHICLE

Drive Hwy 97 ALT, either south from Chelan or north from Wenatchee, to the town of Entiat. Turn west onto the Entiat River Road. At 27.8 mi (44.8 km) pass Lake Creek campground. At 29 mi (46.7 km) turn right onto Road 5900. Pass Halfway Springs at 33.1 mi (53.3 km). At 37.5 mi (60.4 km) reach Shady Pass and turn left onto Road 112. (Do not descend east.) At 38.3 mi (61.6 km) Lake Chelan is visible below. At 39.4 mi (63.4 km) proceed straight on Road 113, ignoring the right fork. Reach the trailhead parking lot at 39.8 mi (64.1 km), 6500 ft (1981 m).

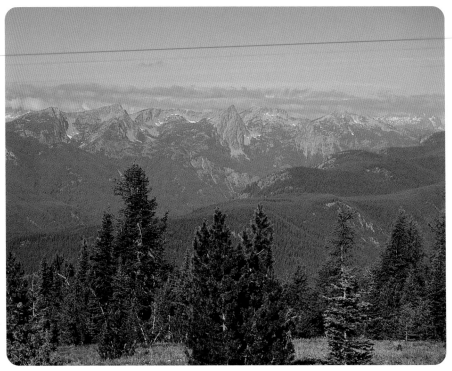

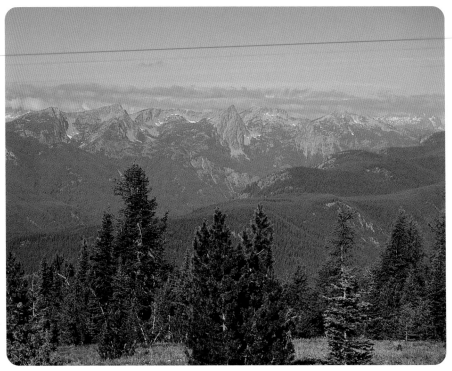

Mt. Maude and Seven Fingered Jack rising above the Entiat River Valley,
from Pyramid Mountain

ON FOOT

Begin following the old road. In 30 yd/m, turn left onto the trail marked by cairns. It switchbacks 0.3 mi (0.5 km) up to rejoin the road. The trail is a bit longer, but it's smoother, easier to walk. Your general direction of travel is west.

After the trail curves north at 0.9 mi (1.4 km), your goal is visible ahead. Pyramid is the bald, rounded mountain on the right. The Entiat Mountains are visible west, beyond the Entiat River valley. Chelan gorge is east, but the lake is obscured. The trees here are tamaracks, or golden larches.

At 1.4 mi (2.3 km), 7000 ft (2134 m) the trail contours along the west side of **Crow Hill**, through grass and lupine. Begin a 600-ft (183-m) switchbacking descent generally northwest at 1.8 mi (2.9 km). At 2.7 mi (4.3 km) reach a junction. The Butte Creek trail forks left (west). Stay right, curving north, descending deeper into forest.

At 3.2 mi (5.1 km) reach the shallow upper reaches of **Butte Creek**. On both sides are pleasant campsites. There's a scattering of wildflowers: pearly everlasting, paintbrush, lupine, and yarrow (numerous tiny white flowers in a clump, atop a stalk with parsley-like leaves).

Beyond forested Butte Creek basin, the trail ascends 600 ft (183 m) in 0.7 mi (1.1 km) via steep switchbacks up the rocky western slope of **Graham Mtn**. The grade then eases. At 4.5 mi (7.2 km) begin a 300-ft (91-m) descent.

At 5.3 mi (8.5 km), from a saddle on the northwest slope of Graham Mtn, you can look east and glimpse Lake Chelan below the Graham Harbor Creek

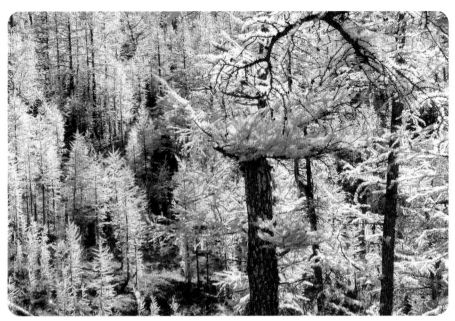

Golden larch

drainage. This is a good rest spot. Just 0.2 mi (0.3 km) farther, you might find a trickle of water in a meadow.

The optimal campsite is at 5.8 mi (9.3 km), in trees beside a level meadow. Proceed through more forest. The trail disappears for 40 yd/m through the next meadow, but continue in the same direction (west) and you'll see it resume on the rocky ascent ahead.

Reach a junction at 6.3 mi (10.1 km), 6800 ft (2073 m). Left descends to Pyramid Creek. Go straight, ascending north. Pyramid Mtn looms closer. Near its base is a small meadow and an unreliable dribble of water. Look in seeps here for magenta elephant's head.

At 7.4 mi (11.9 km) the trail contours left (west)—among clumps of grass, scattered rocks, and whitebark pine—along the south slope of Pyramid Mtn. The final 1.7-mi (2.7-km), 1245-ft (379-m) ascent is via the mellow west slope, instead of the much steeper south slope that was visible during the approach. Moderately graded switchbacks allow you to maintain momentum. Yellow stonecrop and faint-pink spreading phlox brighten the arid terrain.

Reach the 8245-ft (2513-m) summit of **Pyramid Mtn** at 9.2 mi (14.8 km). Directly northwest is the ridge of Cardinal Peak. Pinnacle Mtn is just beyond it. Seven Fingered Jack and Mt. Maude are way northwest. Across the Lake Chelan gorge are mountains of the Lake Chelan-Sawtooth Wilderness.

While surveying Lake Chelan, it's interesting to know that it was dammed in 1927, causing the lake to rise 7 yd/m and gain 1 mi (1.6 km) in length. Much was submerged: natural beaches, homesteads, townsites such as Lakeside, historic resorts such as the Field Hotel, plus Native American rock art and archaeological sites. Ironically, *chelan* is a Native word meaning *deep, beautiful water*.

LYMAN LAKE

LOCATION	Glacier Peak Wilderness / Wenatchee National Forest
ROUND TRIP	18.6 mi (30 km) to Lyman Lake
ELEVATION GAIN	2398 ft (731 m) to Lyman Lake
KEY ELEVATIONS	trailhead 3200 ft (975 m), Hart Lake 3982 ft (1214 m)
	Lyman Lake 5598 ft (1706 m), Cloudy Pass 6438 ft (1962 m)
HIKING TIME	2 to 5 days
DIFFICULTY	moderate
MAP	*Green Trails* Holden 113

OPINION

A boat trip up Lake Chelan and a bus ride to Holden village are your slingshot entry to superb backpacking country. About 2 ½ hours after leaving your vehicle—during which you'll be sightseeing, not sweating—you'll set foot in Railroad Creek valley, where handsome peaks reveal their chiseled profiles within a couple miles.

In the North Cascades, attaining scenery of this magnitude can require a full day's slog. But at Holden, you're already 11 miles (17.7 km) up a mountain canyon. Scenic inspiration is then constant as you follow Railroad Creek upstream. Soon, Hart Lake appears. The slopes northeast of it echo those in Waterton National Park, in Alberta, Canada. To the south is Dumbell Mtn. With its red-orange soil and streaks of alpine greenery, it resembles the leviathans in Colorado's San Juan Wilderness.

Along the way, the forest understory is pleasingly varied. Streams are frequently audible. In early summer, cascades grace the valley walls. And the well-maintained trail allows easy, eyes-on-the-prize striding.

The Lyman Lakes basin is a world apart from the green hues of Railroad Creek below. Hike past turquoise Lyman Lake, into the desolate, Tibetan-like, upper-lakes basin, where Lyman Glacier has chewed away at Chiwawa Mtn. The mosquitoes and black flies will be chewing on you in this bug-infested glacial pocket, so don't camp there.

Ideally, allow yourself three or four days for exploring the wilderness at Holden's back door. Boating up Lake Chelan and backpacking to Lyman Lake are sufficiently rewarding to justify a speedy two-day journey, but an additional couple days allow you to extend the adventure over Cloudy Pass to Image Lake (Trip 44).

Cloudy Pass is an alpine saddle on the shoulder of Cloudy Peak. The pass affords a commanding view of Lyman Lakes and all the mountains ringing them. The trail west to Suiattle Pass and along meadowy Miners Ridge to Image Lake is a North Cascades classic.

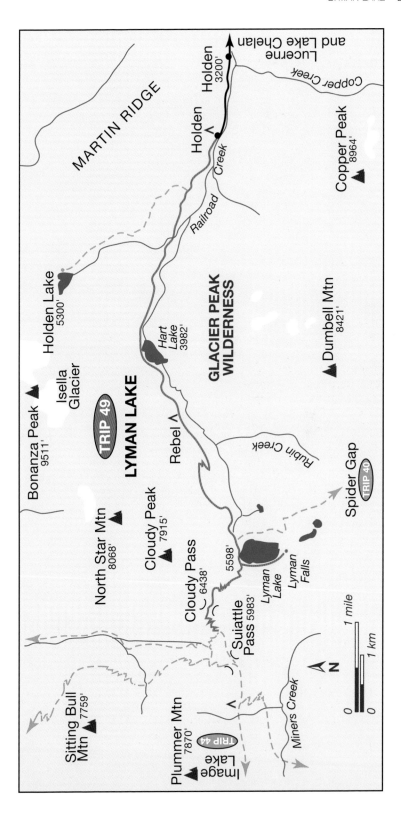

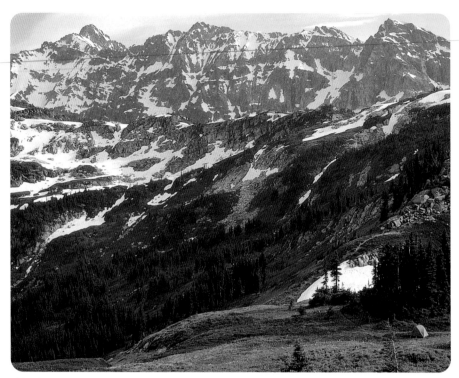

Cloudy Pass

Holden was originally a mining settlement. Copper ore was discovered here in 1896. After production began in 1937, track was laid in Railroad Creek valley with the intention of hauling ore from Holden down to Lucerne. But the railroad was never completed. Instead, the ore was trucked to the barges waiting on Lake Chelan. After the trip down-lake to the town of Chelan, the ore was transported to Tacoma, then shipped to points beyond. Be thankful the rugged topography around Cloudy and Suiattle passes discouraged surveyors from pushing a road west through the mountains. Otherwise this wild valley would now be tame: plowed, paved, and populated.

FACT

BY VEHICLE

Drive to the town of Chelan. It's north of Wenatchee, at the southeast end of Lake Chelan. From there, drive Hwy 971 west along the lakeshore. Pass Chelan State Park on the right. At 17.5 mi (28.2 km), turn right into the Wenatchee National Forest / Lake Chelan National Recreation Area parking lot. This is Fields Point landing. Starting here, rather than in Chelan, the boat trip is 45 minutes shorter. There's a per-night fee for parking here, as there is in Chelan.

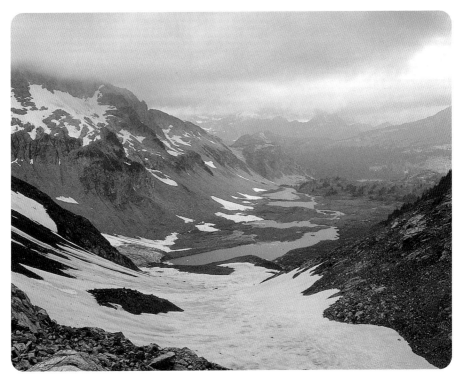

Upper Lyman Lakes, from Spider Gap (Trip 40)

BY BOAT

After departing Fields Point, both the *Lady of the Lake II* and the *Lady Express* stop at Lucerne. Disembark at Lucerne either before or after the boat calls at Stehekin. In advance, tell the purser or the captain where and when you want to get off. From Fields Point, the cruising times are about 2 hours to Lucerne and 2½ hours to Stehekin. For current fares and schedules, visit www.ladyofthelake.com, write to info@ladyofthelake.com, phone (509) 682-4584 to speak to a person, or phone (509) 682-2224 for a recorded message.

During the boat trip, contemplate this: you're in the deepest gorge in the United States. The Grand Canyon is 1 mi (1.6 km) deep. Kings Canyon in California is 7800 ft (2377 m) deep. Hells Canyon on the Idaho/Oregon border is 8200 ft (2500 m) deep. Lake Chelan gorge is deeper still, measuring 8631 ft (2631 m). It was gouged by glaciers 14,000 to 17,000 years ago. Some say Hells Canyon is the deepest, but they're measuring from a highpoint 8 mi (12.9 km) away from the lowpoint along the Snake River. The Lake Chelan gorge is measured from the 8245-ft (2513-m) summit of Pyramid Mtn (Trip 48)—about three-quarters of the way up the lake, on the west side. That high point is only 3 horizontal miles (4.8 km) west from the lowpoint at the bottom of Lake Chelan—386 ft (118 m) below sea level. So Lake Chelan gorge is 431 ft (131 m) deeper than Hells Canyon. After Crater Lake in Oregon, Lake Chelan is the second deepest lake in North America.

Ride the shuttle bus from the Lucerne boat dock, at 1100 ft (335 m), up-canyon, 11 mi (17.7 km) west to Holden, at 3200 ft (975 m).

Now a Lutheran retreat center, Holden once had a population of 600 and served Washington's largest copper mine. When the price of copper plummeted in the 1950s, the mine closed and the village emptied. Unable to sell the village, the mining company donated it to the Lutheran Church.

Visit www.holden.org to learn more about Holden and see the current bus schedule. If you don't intend to stay at the village, visit www.holdenvillage.org/notregistered.html for current bus fares.

Walk the unpaved road west from Holden. It follows Railroad Creek upstream above its north bank. Ignore the bridge spanning the creek. Pass the cement foundations of the long-gone miners' town. At 1 mi (1.6 km) enter Glacier Peak Wilderness. Proceed generally northwest on trail.

Visible directly south is 8964-ft (2732-m) Copper Peak, whose immutable facade belies that it's hollow: honeycombed with 56 miles of tunnels. Copper Peak supplied the lifeblood for the once-thriving miners' town you just passed. Ten million tons of ore were extracted—enough to cover the surface of Lake Chelan. During 20 years of production, that ore was converted into $66.5 million worth of copper, gold and zinc. Now people come to Holden in search of a more enduring form of wealth: spiritual inspiration.

In a forest of cottonwood, mixed conifer and giant willow, ascend to a signed junction at 1.9 mi (3.1 km), 3600 ft (1097 m). Right leads 4 mi (6.4 km) to Holden Lake. Continue straight, contouring northwest. Open forest grants views southwest across the valley to 8421-ft (2567-m) Dumbell Mtn.

At 2.7 mi (4.3 km) cross the bridge spanning Holden Lake's outlet stream. The trail steepens at 3.5 mi (5.6 km) on the lower slopes of 9511-ft (2899-m) Bonanza Peak, the highest non-volcanic summit in Washington.

Reach the northeast end of **Hart Lake** at 4.75 mi (7.6 km), 3982 ft (1214 m). Look for bog orchids and mariposa lilies near the shore. Tentsites here are shaded by cottonwoods. Above the north side of the lake, the trail crosses a stream that can be difficult to ford in early summer.

After a level stretch, pass **Rebel camp** at 5.9 mi (9.5 km). The grade then steepens. At 7 mi (11.3 km) switchback up the Railroad Grade headwall, over which Crown Point Falls plunges. Berries—huckle and blue—are plentiful here in season.

Reach a junction at 9.1 mi (14.6 km), 5500 ft (1676 m). Left (south) rises over a low ridge, enters the fir-and-larch-scattered **upper Lyman Lakes basin** at 6000 ft (1829 m), ascends south-southeast past the Lyman Glacier, then diminishes to a route before cresting Spider Gap at 3 mi (3.8 km), 7100 ft (2164 m), between Dumbell Mtn (left) and Chiwawa Mtn (right). From this side, don't attempt to reach the gap without an ice axe. Hikers scramble to the gap from its south side, via Spider Meadow.

At the 9.1-mi (14.6-km) junction, proceed straight (west-southwest) to reach **Lyman Lake** at 9.3 mi (15 km), 5598 ft (1706 m). It's vastly larger than the upper Lyman Lakes and affords more sheltered camping. At 9.4 mi (15.1 km), reach another junction. Left is a 0.7-mi (1.1-km) spur heading generally south, past tentsites along the lake's west shore, through heather meadows, to the cascading inlet stream and a view of Bonanza Peak (north-northeast). The main trail proceeds straight, soon climbing northwest to reach 6438-ft (1962-m) **Cloudy Pass** at 10.4 mi (16.7 km).

The view from Cloudy Pass, particularly southeast across the Lyman Lakes to Lyman Glacier and the mountains bookending Spider Gap, is a gratifying climax to this trip. Turn around, and 7759-ft (2365-m) Sitting Bull Mtn is visible north-northwest. Walk through the pass for a peek north into South Fork Agnes Creek valley. Two off-trail options lure strong hikers higher for even better views. Head southwest 0.5 mi (0.8 km) for a knoll-top panorama that includes Glacier Peak (southwest). Or ascend higher yet, northeast toward 7915-ft (2412-m) Cloudy Peak.

Beyond Cloudy Pass, the trail begins a switchbacking descent generally southwest to a junction at 10.9 mi (17.5 km), where left leads west-southwest to 5983-ft (1824-m) **Suiattle Pass** at 11.6 mi (18.7 km). Farther west, via trail 785 along Miners Ridge, is **Image Lake** at 15.8 mi (25.4 km).

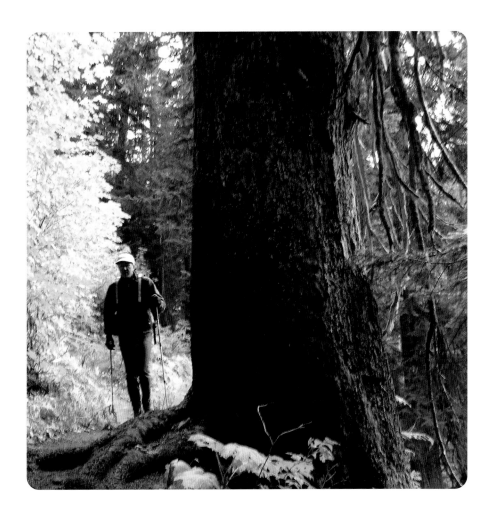

TRIP 50
LAKE CHELAN SHOULDER SEASON

LOCATION	Wenatchee National Forest
	Lake Chelan National Rec Area
ONE-WAY TRIP	17 mi (27.4 km) from Prince Creek to Stehekin
ELEVATION GAIN	2200 ft (671 m)
KEY ELEVATIONS	trailhead / lakeshore 1100 ft (335 m)
	highpoint 1700 ft (518 m)
HIKING TIME	2 to 3 days
DIFFICULTY	easy
MAPS	*Green Trails* Prince Creek 115, Lucerne 114, Stehekin 82

OPINION

The North Cascades are known as *the American Alps*, because they're Swiss in size and appearance. But from the Lake Chelan trail, the range can seem more Greek or Norwegian. Greek because it's often brilliantly sunny and blazing hot here. Norwegian because this isn't a mere mountain lake. It's a fantastic inland fiord.

Welcome to one of the world's great walks. The journey begins with a 20-mi (32.2-km) boat trip up-lake to the Prince Creek trailhead. Continuing north, the trail dances along Lake Chelan's rocky, rugged, Mediterranean-like east shore. You're often within view of the deep, deliciously clear water and the gargantuan mountains that hold it in place.

The most stirring stretch is between Moore Point and Flick Creek, where you'll attain a lake-to-sky spectacle from high on Hunts Bluff. Several tentsites on the north end of Hunts Bluff offer grand views north to Stehekin and south as far as Domke Mtn, but there's no water source nearby.

You'll be about 200 ft (61 m) above the lake most of the way. At several points you'll be within 50 ft (15 m) of the lapping water. For a little less than a third of the total mileage—about 5 mi (8 km)—the trail winds away from the lake into ponderosa-pine forest and lush, creek gorges—cool, moist respites from the arid lakeshore. In damp spots, look for tiger lilies flying on high stems like miniature orange space capsules.

Unless you're a desert rat accustomed to heat, don't hike here between June and September. If you must hike in June, wait for a cool spell, or go right after a rainy period. The mercury can rise to 105°F (41°C) by mid May, and the steep shoreline makes it difficult to cool off in the water as often as you might like.

The lake's popularity with boaters is another reason to hike here in early spring. The later you come, the more boaters you'll have to share the campgrounds with. This is rattlesnake country too, so be alert. Also check yourself thoroughly for ticks at rest stops and at day's end.

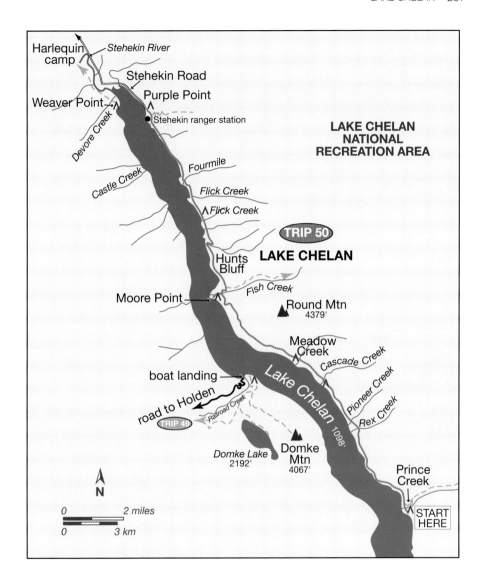

Harlequin camp
Stehekin River
Stehekin Road
Purple Point
Weaver Point
Stehekin ranger station
Devore Creek
Castle Creek
Fourmile
Flick Creek
Flick Creek
TRIP 50
Hunts Bluff
LAKE CHELAN NATIONAL RECREATION AREA
LAKE CHELAN
Fish Creek
Moore Point
Round Mtn 4379'
Meadow Creek
Cascade Creek
Pioneer Creek
boat landing
Lake Chelan 1098'
Rex Creek
road to Holden
Railroad Creek
TRIP 49
Domke Lake 2192'
Domke Mtn 4067'
Prince Creek
N
0   2 miles
0   3 km
START HERE

Strong hikers who disembark at Prince Creek around 11 a.m. can cover the 11 mi (17.7 km) to Moore Point for the first night's camp. The Meadow Creek campsites at 7 mi (11.3 km) are less appealing. If you reach Moore Point the first day, you can finish the hike the next day in time to catch the boat departing from Stehekin at about 2 p.m. for its down-lake journey. If you only want to dayhike, disembark at Moore Point and walk the 6.8 mi (10.9 km) north to Stehekin. You can arrange to leave gear on the boat and have it dropped at Stehekin Landing. In Stehekin, you can camp at Purple Point or stay in one of the lodges.

To fully appreciate the deepest gorge in the U.S., hike the Chelan Lakeshore in spring, then come back after July and hike to the top of Pyramid Mtn (Trip 48). From there you can look straight down at the lake, 7145 ft (2178 m) below, and see just how colossal the surrounding mountains really are.

FACT

Drive to the town of Chelan. It's north of Wenatchee, at the southeast end of Lake Chelan. From there, drive Hwy 971 west along the lakeshore. Pass Chelan State Park on the right. At 17.5 mi (28.2 km), turn right into the Wenatchee National Forest / Lake Chelan National Recreation Area parking lot. This is Fields Point landing. Starting here, rather than in Chelan, the boat trip is 45 minutes shorter. There's a per-night fee for parking here, as there is in Chelan.

To disembark at Prince Creek, where the trail begins, hikers must take the slower boat: the *Lady of the Lake II.* From Fields Point, the cruising times are about 1½ hours to Prince Creek, 2 hours to Lucerne, and 2½ hours to Stehekin.

If you want to hike the trails out of Holden, as well as the lakeshore, it's logical to hike the lakeshore first. Then, on the down-lake boat trip, disembark at Lucerne to catch the bus to Holden. Wherever you decide to get off, tell the purser or the captain in advance.

For current fares and schedules, visit www.ladyofthelake.com, write to info@ladyofthelake.com, phone (509) 682-4584 to speak to a person, or phone (509) 682-2224 for a recorded message.

During the boat trip, contemplate this: you're in the deepest gorge in the United States. The Grand Canyon is 1 mi (1.6 km) deep. Kings Canyon in California is 7800 ft (2377 m) deep. Hells Canyon on the Idaho/Oregon border is 8200 ft (2500 m) deep. Lake Chelan gorge is deeper still, measuring 8631 ft (2631 m). It was gouged by glaciers 14,000 to 17,000 years ago. Some say Hells Canyon is the deepest, but they're measuring from a highpoint 8 mi (12.9 km) away from the lowpoint along the Snake River. The Lake Chelan gorge is measured from the 8245-ft (2513-m) summit of Pyramid Mtn (Trip 48)—about three-quarters of the way up the lake, on the west side. That high point is only 3 horizontal miles (4.8 km) west from the lowpoint at the bottom of Lake Chelan—386 ft (118 m) below sea level. So Lake Chelan gorge is 431 ft (131 m) deeper than Hells Canyon. After Crater Lake in Oregon, Lake Chelan is the second deepest lake in North America.

The boat drops hikers either north or south of **Prince Creek**, at 1100 ft (335 m). The following distances start at the campground immediately south of the creek. Your general direction of travel will remain northwest all the way to Moore Point junction.

The trail crosses the Prince Creek alluvial fan. The creek is bridged. There's another campground 0.1 mi (0.2 km) north of the creek, in meadows and ponderosa pines, where the creek is more audible. At 0.3 mi (0.5 km) ignore the Prince Creek trail. It forks right, heading upstream to Cub Lake. Soon after, the lakeshore trail gains 200 ft (61 m).

The trail is often level, but has some short, steep climbs. At 3 mi (4.8 km)—where you can see Domke Falls west across the lake—there's a very

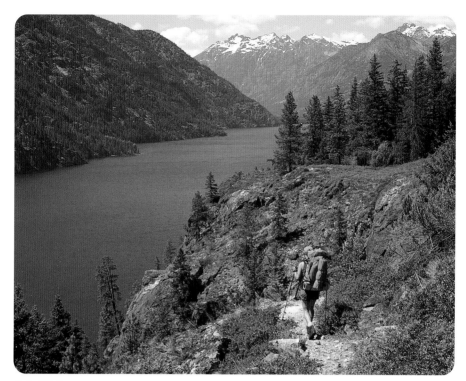

Lake Chelan

steep ascent. The trail then descends to an easy ford of **Rex Creek** at 3.5 mi (5.6 km). The next ford, **Pioneer Creek**, can be difficult after heavy rain. Beyond it is a 0.25-mi (0.4-km) flat area where you could pitch a tent in the trees. Domke Mtn dominates the western horizon across the lake for a long stretch. Cross **Cascade Creek** near 6.25 mi (10.1 km).

At 7.7 mi (12.4 km) reach the lush environs of **Meadow Creek**. Just below the Meadow Creek shelter are a couple tentsites among scruffy pines. Private property here makes it difficult to access the lake or find an attractive campsite, especially after dusk. To do so, proceed 0.7 mi (1.1 km) past the shelter, then cut left off the trail and walk cross-country toward the lakeshore. Descend 150 ft (46 m) in 0.2 mi (0.3 km). Look for a flat spot among ponderosa pines on a bench above the lake.

After a long, gradual ascent, partly on an old road, the main trail reaches its 1700-ft (518-m) highpoint at 9.7 mi (15.6 km). A view north opens up. Descend steep switchbacks generally west, before turning north again. After passing a broad meadow, reach **Moore Point junction** on the south side of the Fish Creek bridge at 10.7 mi (17.2 km).

The main trail proceeds straight, across the bridge. Your general direction of travel will remain north-northwest all the way to Stehekin. To reach **Moore Point camp**, turn left and hike downstream. From the Fish Creek bridge, the spur descends west-southwest 0.5-mi (0.8-km) to the lake at 1100 ft (335 m).

In 1889 the upper lake's first hotel was built here on an alluvial fan. During a catastrophic region-wide flood in 1948, Fish Creek raged across the

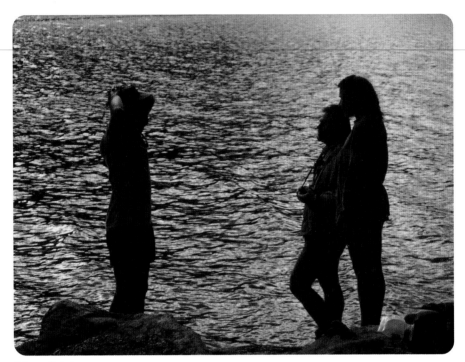

Moore Point

fan, dragging pieces of the hotel with it. That was the end of business. The rest of the building burned in 1957. Stone walls around a pasture are all that remain. Moore Point is now a large Forest Service campground offering a rough shelter, tables, toilets, fire pits, and space for numerous tents. Boaters often claim the lakeshore sites before hikers arrive. Fish Creek is audible even from the most distant campsites at the south end.

Continuing north on the main trail from Moore Point junction, cross the **Fish Creek bridge**. After ascending 200 ft (61 m) in 0.4 mi (0.6 km), pass the Fish Creek trail. It forks right, following the creek upstream (west). Just north of that junction, there's a potentially confusing network of old roads. At a seeming fork near a creek, stay right and go toward the creek. Don't follow the broad, descending road. Look for the sign pointing north to Stehekin and south to Prince Creek.

After ascending a rocky traverse (not precarious), crest **Hunts Bluff** at 12.2 mi (19.6 km), 1600 ft (488 m). Views are expansive south, down-lake to Pinnacle Mtn.

Gradually descend, crossing **Hunts Creek**, then an unnamed stream. Just after private property ends, enter the National Recreation Area at 13.3 mi (21.4 km). For the next 0.4 mi (0.7 km), the trail is about 7 yd/m above the water. **Flick Creek campground** is on the lakeshore at 13.7 mi (22 km). It's small, with room for only a couple tents. It also has a shelter, a table, and a toilet.

Beyond Flick Creek the trail is beneath cliffs, about 100 ft (30 m) above the water. It darts in and out of forest. Cross Flick Creek at 14.5 mi (23.3 km), then bridged **Fourmile Creek** at 15.2 mi (24.5 km). Just past Fourmile is a campsite in trees overlooking the lake. It could be handy if Flick is full. The trail makes a couple ascents around rock outcroppings. Lake views are frequent the remaining distance to Stehekin. Pass private summer homes just before **Hazard Creek** and a waterfall at 16.7 mi (26.9 km).

Arrive in **Stehekin** 17 mi (27.4 km) from Prince Creek. You'll first see the North Cascades Lodge and a sign for overflow camping. It has numerous tentsites, two toilets, and a water faucet up-slope behind the ranger station.

To reach **Purple Point campground** in Stehekin, continue 0.4 mi (0.6 km) north. It can be difficult to find the trail that contours the hillside, so just walk the lakeshore road through Stehekin. Pass the ranger station, the visitor center, and the visitor services at the boat landing. The campground is just north of Purple Creek. It has tables, firepits, toilets, and several tentsites well-separated in the woods. The sites are above the infrequently used road and across from buildings. Views of the lake and mountains are obscured. A shower and laundry is just south of the campground. To camp at Purple Point, get a free permit from the Golden West visitor center in Stehekin.

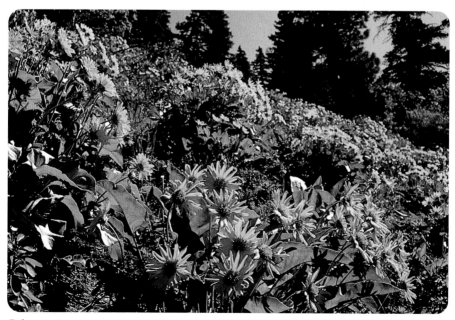

Balsamroot

PREPARE FOR YOUR HIKE

Hiking in the North Cascades is an adventure. Adventure involves risk. But the rewards are worth it. Just be ready for more adventure than you expect. The weather here is constantly changing. Even on a warm, sunny day, pack for rain or snow. Injury is always a possibility. On a long dayhike, be equipped to spend the night out. If you respect the power of wilderness by being prepared, you'll decrease the risk, increase your comfort and enjoyment, and come away fulfilled, yearning for more.

The following recommendations will help you know what's best to pack for mountain conditions. If you don't own or can't afford some of the gear listed, make do with what you have. Just be sure to bring warm clothing that insulates when wet. Cotton is terrible. Merino superfine wool and synthetics like Capilene are much better. Visit www.sierratradingpost.com, an online outlet store used by most of North America's leading outdoor gear manufacturers to blow out remaindered stock.

YOU CARRY WHAT YOU ARE

Even with all the right gear, you're ill-equipped without physical fitness. If the weather turns grim, the physical capability to escape the wilderness fast might keep you from being stuck in a life-threatening situation. If you're fit, and a companion gets injured, you can race for help. Besides, if you're not overweight or easily exhausted, you'll have more fun. You'll be able to hike farther, reach more spectacular scenery, and leave crowds behind. So if you're out of shape, work on it. Everything else you'll need is easier to acquire.

TRAVEL LIGHT

Weight is critical when backpacking. The lighter you travel, the easier and more pleasant the journey. Carrying too much can sour your opinion of an otherwise great trip. Some people are mules; they can shoulder everything they want. If you'd rather be a thoroughbred, reduce your load and get lighter gear. You might have to sacrifice a little luxury at the campsite in order to be more agile, fleet-footed and comfortable on the trail, but you'll be a happier hiker.

Weigh your pack when it's empty. Switching to a newer, lighter model might shave a couple pounds off your burden. A palatial dome tent is probably overdoing it. Check out the smaller, lighter, anthropomorphic designs. A down sleeping bag will weigh less, stuff smaller and last longer than a synthetic-filled bag that has the same temperature rating. You can also cut weight and volume with a ¾ -length inflatable sleeping-pad instead of a full-length one made of thick foam. Forget that heavy, bulky, fleece jacket. If you get really cold at camp, wear your raingear over other, insulating layers. And on any trek less than four days, it's possible to pack only real food and leave all that clunky cooking equipment at home. Try it. Hot meals aren't necessary. Playing outdoor chef and dishwasher is a time-consuming ordeal. It also makes it harder to leave no trace of your visit, and it can attract bears. Select the right foods and you'll find they weigh no more than a stove, fuel, pots, and pre-packaged meals.

These reductions long ago revitalized our interest in backpacking. Now we revel in going light. Lighter equipment is more expensive because the materials are finer quality and the craftsmanship superior. But it's definitely worth it. Consult reputable outdoor stores for specific brands.

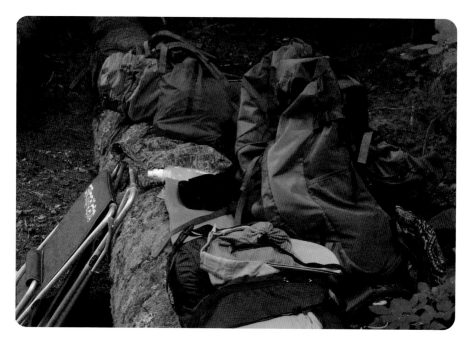

UNNECESSARY STUFF

We once encountered two men laboring up a North Cascades trail, bound for a distant, backcountry lake, pushing wheelbarrows piled with camping "necessities." They had a cooler, tackle box, hatchet, lawn chairs, even a radio. They also had sore hands, aching spines, and a new appreciation for backpacks and minimal loads.

Unless you're in terrific shape, have a high pain threshold, or don't mind creeping along at a slug's pace, think about everything you pack. Jettisoning preconceptions will lighten your burden.

You don't need the entire guidebook. Take notes, or photocopy the pages of your book. Carrying the whole thing is like lugging a rock in your pack. Even an iPod is questionable, and not just because of the added weight. Toting tunes into the outdoors will deny you the delight of birdsong, windsong, riversong. Wearing headphones blunts your awareness, increasing the likelihood of a bear encounter.

An extra pair of shoes? No way. Even sandals are heavy. For in-camp comfort, bring a pair of beach flip-flops. The cheap, $1.99 variety are almost weightless, and their treadless soles are easy on the environment.

Jeans are ridiculous. They're heavy, restrictive, and don't insulate. Cotton sweatpants are almost as bad. Anything 100% cotton is a mistake, as explained below.

LAYER WITH SYNTHETICS

Don't just wear a T-shirt and throw a heavy sweatshirt in your pack. Cotton kills. It quickly gets saturated with perspiration and takes way too long to dry. Wet clothing saps your body heat and could lead to hypothermia, a leading cause of death in the outdoors. Your mountain clothes should be made of synthetic fabrics that wick sweat away from your skin, insulate when wet, and dry rapidly. Even your hiking shorts and underwear should be at least partly synthetic. Sports bras should be entirely synthetic.

There are now lots of alternatives to the soggy T-shirt. All outdoor clothing companies offer shortsleeve shirts in superior, synthetic versions. Unlike cotton T-shirts, sweat-soaked synthetics can dry during a rest break.

For warmth, several synthetic layers are more efficient than a single parka. Your body temperature varies constantly on the trail, in response to the weather and your activity level. With only one warm garment, it's either on or off, roast or freeze. Layers allow you to fine tune for optimal comfort.

In addition to a synthetic shortsleeve shirt, it's smart to pack two longsleeve tops (zip-T's) of different fabric weights: one thin, one thick. Wear the thin one for cool-weather hiking. It'll be damp when you stop for a break, so change into the thick one. When you start again, put the thin one back on. The idea is to always keep your thick top dry in case you really need it to stay warm. Covered by a rain shell (jacket), these two tops can provide enough warmth on summer hikes. You can always wear your shortsleeve shirt like a vest over a longsleeve top. For more warmth on the trail, try a fleece vest. For more warmth in camp, consider a down vest or down sweater. But don't hike in down clothing; it'll get sweat soaked and become useless.

For your legs, bring a pair of tights or long underwear, both if you're going overnight. Choose tights made of synthetic insulating material, with a small percentage of lycra for stretchiness. These are warmer and more durable than the all-lycra or nylon/lycra tights runners wear. Tights are generally more efficient than pants. They stretch, conforming to your movement. They're lighter and insulate better. You can wear them for hours in a drizzle and not feel damp. If you're too modest to sport this sleek look, just wear shorts over them. Shorts also protect tights from snagging when you sit down.

Anticipating hot weather? Mosquitoes? Exposure to intense sun? You'll want long pants and a longsleeve shirt, both made of tightly-woven synthetics and as lightweight as possible. Make sure they fit loosely enough to be unrestrictive. The shirt should resemble a dress shirt—collar, button front, cuffs—but be designed specifically for vigorous activity. Most outdoor clothing manufacturers offer them. They're pricey, of course. So if you want a bargain version, visit your local used-clothing store and buy a mostly-synthetic dress shirt or blouse for a couple bucks. And if you have the confidence and sense of humour to flaunt your frugal practicality, pick one in a color and pattern that screams "fashion-challenged corporate executive."

RAINGEAR

Pack a full set of raingear: shell and pants. The shell (jacket) should have a hood. Fabrics that are both waterproof and breathable are best, because they repel rain *and* vent perspiration vapor. Gore-tex has long been the fabric of choice, but there are now many alternatives—equally effective, yet less expensive.

Don't let a blue sky or a promising weather forecast tempt you to leave your raingear behind. It can be invaluable, even if you don't encounter rain. Worn over insulating layers, a shell and pants will shed wind, retain body heat, and keep you much warmer.

Coated-nylon raingear might appear to be a bargain, but it doesn't breathe, so it simulates a steam bath if worn while exercising. You'll end up as

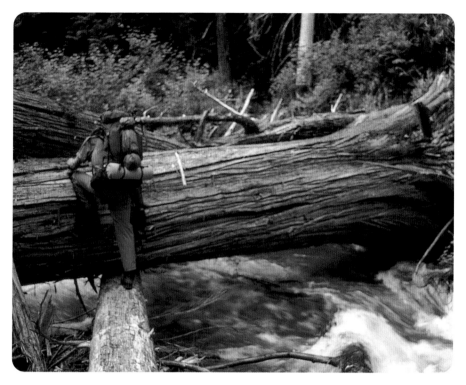

damp from sweat as you would from rain. You're better off with a poncho, if you can't afford technical raingear. On a blustery day, a poncho won't provide impervious protection from rain, but at least it will allow enough air circulation so you won't get sweat soaked.

BOOTS AND SOCKS

Lightweight fabric boots with even a little ankle support are more stable and safer than runners. But all-leather or highly technical leather/fabric boots offer superior comfort and performance. For serious hiking, they're a necessity. Here are a few points to remember while shopping for boots.

If it's a rugged, quality boot, a light- or medium-weight pair should be adequate for most hiking conditions. Heavy boots will slow you down, just like an overweight pack. But you want boots with hard, protective toes, or you'll risk a broken or sprained digit.

Lateral support stops ankle injuries. Stiff shanks keep your feet from tiring. Grippy outsoles prevent slipping and falling. And sufficient cushioning lessens the pain of a long day on the trail.

Out of the box, boots should be waterproof or at least very water resistant, although you'll have to treat them often to retain their repellency. Boots with lots of seams allow water to seep in as they age. A full rand (wrap-around bumper) adds an extra measure of water protection.

The key consideration is comfort. Make sure your boots don't hurt. If you wait to find out until after a day of hiking, it's too late; you're stuck with them. So before handing over your cash, ask the retailer if, after wearing them in a shopping mall, you can exchange them if they don't feel right. A half-hour of mall walking is a helpful test.

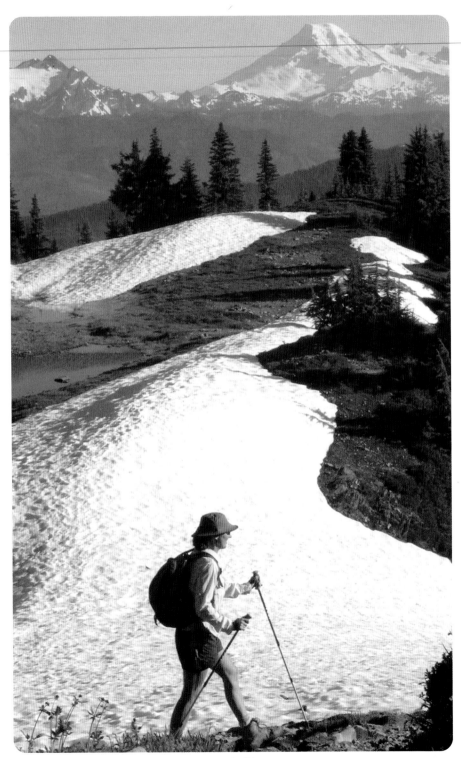

Trekking poles could add years to your mountain life.

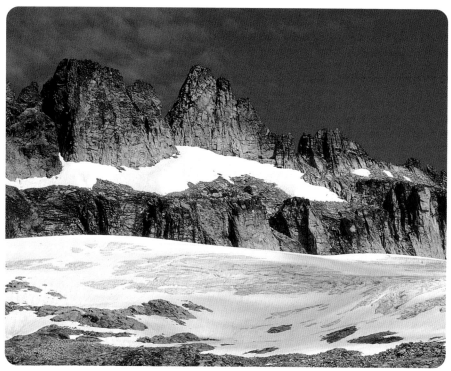

Above Boston Basin

Socks are important too. To keep your feet dry, warm and happy, wear wool, thick acrylic, or wool/acrylic-blend socks. Cotton socks retain sweat, cause blisters, and are especially bad if your boots aren't waterproof. It's usually best to wear two pairs of socks, with a thinner, synthetic pair next to your feet to wick away moisture and alleviate friction, minimizing the chance of blisters.

GLOVES AND HATS

Always bring gloves and a hat. You've probably heard it, and it's true: your body loses most of its heat through your head and extremities. Cover them if you get chilled. Carry thin, synthetic gloves to wear while hiking. Don't worry if they get wet, but keep a pair of thicker fleece gloves dry in your pack. A fleece hat, or at least a thick headband that covers your ears, adds a lot of warmth and weighs little. A hat with a long brim is essential to shade your eyes and protect your face from sun exposure.

TREKKING POLES

Long, steep ascents and descents in the North Cascades make trekking poles vital. Hiking with poles is easier, more enjoyable, and less punishing to your body. If you're constantly pounding the trails, they could add years to your mountain life.

Working on a previous guidebook, we once hiked for a month without poles. Both of us developed knee pain. The next summer we used Leki

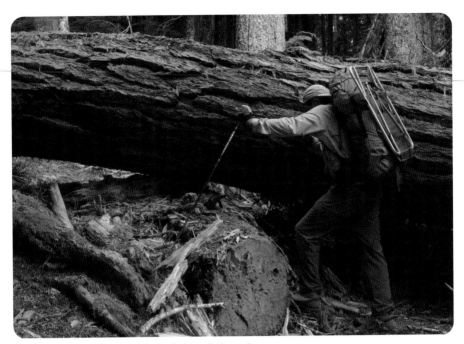

Deadfall is a frequent obstacle in the North Cascades.

trekking poles every day for three months and our knees were never strained. We felt like four-legged animals. We were more sure-footed. Our speed and endurance increased.

Studies show that during a typical 8-hour hike you'll transfer more than 250 tons of pressure to a pair of trekking poles. When going downhill, poles significantly reduce stress to your knees, as well as your ankles and lower back. They alleviate knee strain when you're going uphill too, because you're climbing with your arms and shoulders, not just your legs. Poles also improve your posture. They keep you more upright, which gives you greater lung capacity and allows more efficient breathing.

The heavier your pack, the more you'll appreciate the support of trekking poles. You'll find them especially helpful for crossing unbridged streams, traversing steep slopes, and negotiating muddy, rooty, rough stretches of trail. Poles prevent ankle sprains—a common hiking injury. By making you more stable, they actually help you relax, boosting your sense of security and confidence.

Don't carry one of those big, heavy, gnarled, wooden staffs, unless you're going to a costume party dressed as Gandalf. They're more burden than benefit. If you can't afford trekking poles, make do with a pair of old ski poles. They're not as effective or comfortable as poles designed specifically for trekking, but they're better than hiking empty handed. If possible, invest in a pair of true trekking poles with a soft anti-shock system and adjustable, telescoping, super-lock shafts. We strongly recommend Lekis.

When backpacking, protect your trekking poles by keeping them inside your tent at night. Otherwise, the grips and straps—salty from your perspiration—will attract critters, such as porcupines, who will quickly chew them to shreds.

FIRST AID

Someone in your hiking party should carry a first-aid kit. Pre-packaged kits look handy, but they're expensive, and some are inadequate. If you make your own, you'll be more familiar with the contents. Include an anti-bacterial ointment; pain pills with ibuprofen, and a few with codeine for agonizing injuries; regular bandages; several sizes of butterfly bandages; a couple bandages big enough to hold a serious laceration together; rolls of sterile gauze and absorbent pads to staunch bleeding; adhesive tape; tiny fold-up scissors or a small knife; and a compact first-aid manual. Whether your kit is store bought or homemade, check the expiration dates on your medications every year and replace them as needed.

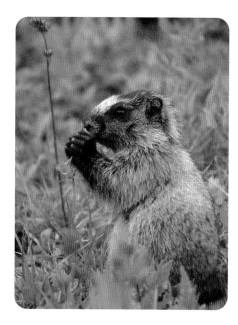

Instead of the old elastic bandages for wrapping sprains, we now carry neoprene ankle and knee bands. They slip on instantly, require no special wrapping technique, keep the injured joint warmer, and stay in place better. They're so convenient, you can quickly slip them on for extra support on long, steep, rough descents.

BANDANAS

A bandana will be the most versatile item in your pack. You can use it to blow your nose, mop your brow, or improvise a beanie. It makes a colorful headband that will keep sweat or hair out of your eyes. It serves as a bandage or sling in a medical emergency. Worn as a neckerchief, it prevents a sunburned neck. If you soak it in water, then drape it around your neck, it will help keep you from overheating. Worn Lawrence-of-Arabia style under a hat, it shades both sides of your face, as well as your neck, while deterring mosquitoes. For an air-conditioning effect, soak it in water then don it á la Lawrence. When shooing away mosquitoes, flicking a bandana with your wrist is less tiresome than flailing your arms. For all these reasons and more, carry at least two bandanas when dayhiking, more when backpacking.

SMALL AND ESSENTIAL

Take matches in a plastic bag, so they'll stay dry. It's wise to carry a lighter, too. Finger-sized fire starters, such as Optimus Firelighter or Coghlan FireSticks, might help you start a fire in an emergency when everything is wet.

Pack an emergency survival bag on dayhikes. One fits into the palm of your hand and could help you survive a cold night without a sleeping bag or tent. The ultralight, metallic fabric reflects your body heat back at you. Survival bags, which you crawl into, are more efficient than survival blankets.

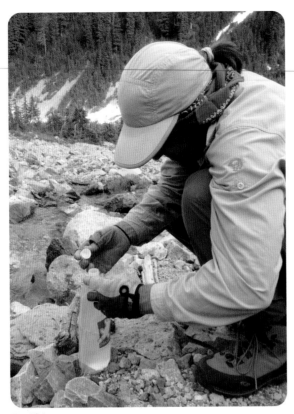

Purifying water

Also bring several plastic bags in various sizes. Use the small ones for packing out garbage. A couple large trash bags could be used to improvise a shelter.

A headlamp is often helpful and can be necessary for safety. You'll need one to stay on the trail if a crisis forces you to hike at night. Carry extra batteries.

Most people find mosquito repellent indispensable. If you anticipate an infestation, bring a head net made of fine, nylon mesh.

For those dreaded blisters, pack Moleskin or Spenco gel. Cut it with the knife or scissors you should have in your first-aid kit.

Wear sunglasses for protection against glare and wind. A few hours in the elements can strain your eyes and even cause a headache. People who don't wear sunglasses are more prone to cataracts later in life. Also bring sunscreen and a hat with a brim. High-altitude sun can fry you fast.

And don't forget to pack lots of thought-provoking questions to ask your companions. Hiking stimulates meaningful conversation.

KEEP IT ALL DRY

Most daypacks and backpacks are not waterproof, or even very water resistant. To protect your gear from rain, put it in plastic bags and use a waterproof pack cover. Rain is a constant likelihood, so you might as well start hiking with everything in bags. That's easier than wrestling with it in a storm. For added assurance, lightweight, waterproof stuffsacks are superior to plastic bags.

WATER

Drink water frequently. Keeping your body hydrated is essential. If you're thirsty, you're probably not performing at optimal efficiency. But be aware of giardia lamblia, a waterborne parasitic cyst that causes severe gastrointestinal distress. It's transported through animal and human feces, so never defecate or urinate near water. To be safe, assume giardia is present in all surface water in the North Cascades. Don't drink any water unless it's directly from a source you're certain is pure, like meltwater dripping off glacial ice, or until you've boiled, disinfected or filtered it.

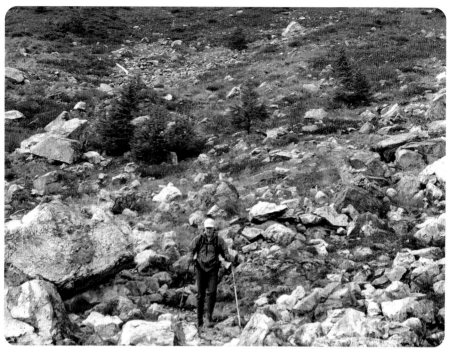

Basin beneath Yellow Aster Butte

Boiling water is a time-consuming hassle, especially along the trail, before reaching your campsite. Boiling also requires you to carry a stove and extra fuel, making it the heaviest method of ensuring safe water.

Killing giardia by disinfecting it with iodine tablets can be tricky. The colder the water, the longer you must wait. Iodine also makes the water smell and taste awful, unless you use neutralizing pills. And iodine has no effect whatsoever on cryptosporidium, an increasingly common cyst that causes physical symptoms identical to giardiasis.

Carrying a small, lightweight filter is a reasonable solution. Some filters weigh just 8 ounces (240 grams). To strain out giardia cysts, your filter must have an absolute pore size of 4 microns or less. Straining out cryptosporidium cysts requires an absolute pore size of 2 microns or less.

After relying on water filters for many years, we've switched to Pristine water purification droplets (www.pristine.ca). The active ingredient is chlorine dioxide, which has been used for more than 50 years in hundreds of water treatment plants throughout North America and Europe. The Pristine system comprises two 30-ml bottles with a total combined weight of only 2.8 ounces (80 grams). It purifies up to 30 gallons (120 litres) of water. Using it is simple: mix two solutions, wait five minutes, then add it to your water. You can drink 15 minutes later knowing you won't contract giardia. Treating for cryptosporidium requires a higher dosage and/or longer wait.

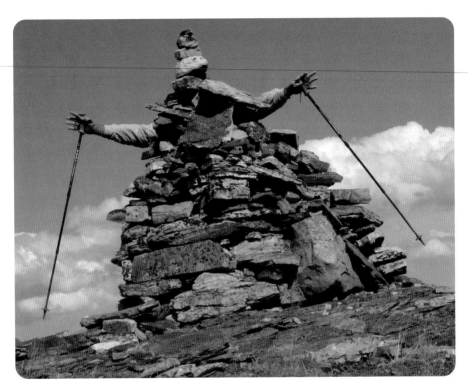

BODY FUEL

When planning meals, keep energy and nutrition foremost in mind. During a six-hour hike, you'll burn 1800 to 3000 calories, depending on terrain, pace, body size, and pack weight. You'll be stronger, and therefore safer and happier, if you tank up on high-octane body fuel.

A white-flour bun with a thick slab of meat or cheese on it is low-octane fuel. Too much protein or fat will make you feel sluggish and drag you down. And you won't get very far up the trail snacking on candy bars. Refined sugars give you a brief spurt that quickly fizzles.

For sustained exercise, like hiking, you need protein and fat to function normally and give you that satisfying full feeling. The speed of your metabolism determines how much protein and fat you should eat. Both are hard to digest. Your body takes three or four hours to assimilate them, compared to one or two hours for carbohydrates. That's why a carb-heavy diet is optimal for hiking. It ensures your blood supply keeps hustling oxygen to your legs, instead of being diverted to your stomach. Most people, however, can sustain athletic effort longer if their carb-heavy diet includes a little protein. So eat a small portion of protein in the morning, a smaller portion at lunch, and a moderate portion at dinner to aid muscle repair.

For athletic performance, the American and Canadian Dietetic Association recommends that 60 to 65% of your total energy come from carbs, less than 25% from fat, and 15% from protein. They also say refined carbs and sugars should account for no more than 10% of your total carb calories.

Toiling muscles crave the glycogen your body manufactures from complex carbs. Yet your body has limited carb storage capacity. So your carb intake should be constant. That means loading your pack with plant foods made of whole-grain flour, rice, corn, oats, legumes, nuts, seeds, fruit and vegetables.

DINING OUT

Natural- or health-food stores are reliable sources of hiking food. They even stock energy bars, which are superior to candy bars because they contain more carbs and less fat. Whether dayhiking or backpacking, always bring extra energy bars for emergencies. We rely on Power Bars. They energize us faster and sustain us longer than any other brand we've tried.

On dayhikes, carry fresh or dried fruit; whole-grain pita bread filled with tabouli, hummus, avocado, cucumbers and sprouts; whole-grain cookies made with natural sweeteners (brown-rice syrup, organic cane-sugar, fruit juice, raw honey); whole-grain crackers; or a bag of organic tortilla chips (corn or mixed-grain) cooked in expeller-pressed safflower or canola oil. Take marinated tofu that's been pressed, baked, and vacuum-packed. It's protein rich, delicious, and lasts about three days. Omnivores have other excellent protein options: hard-boiled eggs, free-range bison jerky, and vacuum-packed wild salmon in a tear-open bag. Don't rely solely on cheese for protein; beyond small amounts, it's unhealthy.

For a backpacking breakfast, spread butter, maple syrup and cinnamon on whole-grain bread, or in pita pockets. Or why not whole-grain cookies in the morning? They're like cereal, only more convenient. The backpacking lunch menu is the same as for dayhiking. For dinner, try bean salad, rice with stir-fried veggies, or pasta with steamed veggies and dressing, all cooked at home and sealed in plastic. Bean burritos made ahead of time, then eaten cold on the trail, are great too. Fresh veggies that travel well include carrots and bell peppers.

For a one- or two-night trip, don't adhere blindly to tradition. Carry a stove only if cooking significantly increases your enjoyment. Real meals are heavier than pre-packaged, but they make up for it by eliminating the weight of cooking equipment and the bother of cooking and cleaning. Plus they're tastier, more filling, cheaper, and better for you. Fresh food tends to be too heavy, bulky and perishable for trips longer than three days. Then it makes sense to pack a stove and dehydrated food. Fast-and-easy options are soup mixes, lentils, and quick-cooking pasta or brown rice.

The best tasting, most nutritious pre-packaged meals we've found are made by Mary Jane's Farm: www.backcountryfood.org. They're dehydrated, so they retain more nutritional value than freeze-dried food. Mary Jane's wide range of delicious soups, pan breads, and dinners (pasta- or grain-based) have kept us from yearning for grocery stores and restaurants, even after a week on the trail. For breakfast, we recommend Mary Jane's *Outrageous Outback Oatmeal*. For dinner, each of us eats a soup as well as a main course. While visiting her website, read Mary Jane's life story. It's both interesting and inspiring. She was one of the first female wilderness rangers in the U.S. She later homesteaded, became an organic farmer, then created her organic backpacking food company.

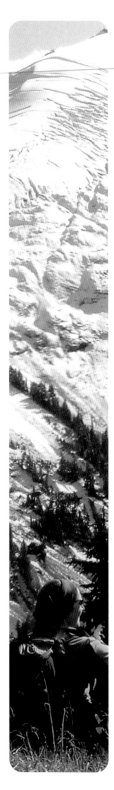

INFORMATION SOURCES

Maps and current trail reports are available at these offices. National Forest offices and ranger stations are usually open from 8 a.m. to 4 p.m. weekdays year-round, with extended hours and days from late-May to mid-September. Check out the Forest Service website (www.fs.fed.us/r6), or North Cascades NP website (www.nps.gov/noca) for details.

TO REPORT A FOREST FIRE, phone (800) 562-6010/1

Mountaineering Search & Rescue, phone 911

Cathedral Provincial Park
ph: (250) 494-6500 / www.bcparks.com
B.C. Parks Regional Office
102 Industrial Place, Penticton, BC V2A 7C8

Chelan Ranger District
ph: (509) 682-2576
Route 2, 428 West Woodin Avenue
Chelan, WA 98816

Darrington Ranger Station
ph: (360) 436-1155 for Glacier Peak Wilderness
1405 Emmens Street
Darrington, WA 98241

Glacier Public Service Center
ph: (360) 599-2714
1094 Mt. Baker Highway 542
Glacier, WA 98244

Lake Chelan National Recreation Area
Golden West Visitor Center
Stehekin District
ph: (360) 856-5703, ext 14 or 340
P.O. Box 7, Stehekin, WA 98852

Lake Wenatchee Ranger Station
ph: (509) 763-3103
22976 State Highway 207
Leavenworth, WA 98826

Manning Provincial Park
ph: (250) 840-8708 / www.bcparks.ca
Visitor Center, Hwy 3, British Columbia

Methow Valley Ranger District
ph: (509) 996-4003
24 West Chewuch
Winthrop, WA 98862

Mt. Baker Ranger District - North Cascades
ph: (360) 856-5700 / www.fs.fed.us/r6/mbs
2105 State Route 20
Sedro Woolley, WA 98284

North Cascades National Park
ph: (206) 386-4495
Visitor Center just off Hwy 20
Newhalem, WA 98283

North Cascades National Park - Wilderness Office
ph: (360) 873-4500, ext 39
7280 Ranger Station Road
Marblemount, WA 98267
Turn off Route 20 at milepost 105.3 in Marblemount.

Okanogan National Forest
ph: (509) 664-9200
215 Melody Lane
Wenatchee, WA 98801

Ross Lake Resort (water-taxi reservations)
ph: (206) 386-4437
www.rosslakeresort.com
Rockport, WA 98283

Tonasket Ranger Station
ph: (509) 486-2186
One West Winesap
Tonasket, WA 98855

Verlot Public Service Center
ph: (360) 691-7791
33515 Mountain Loop Hwy
Granite Falls, WA 98252

Washington Trails Association
ph: (206) 625-1367 / www.wta.org
2019 Third Avenue, Suite 100
Seattle, WA 98121

Washington Weather
www.wsdot.wa.gov/traffic/weather

Wenatchee National Forest
ph: (509) 664-9200
215 Melody Lane
Wenatchee, WA 98801

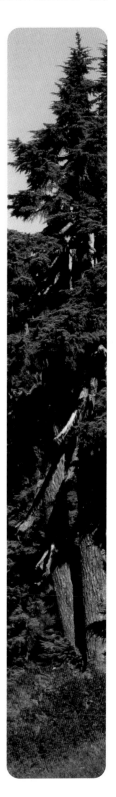

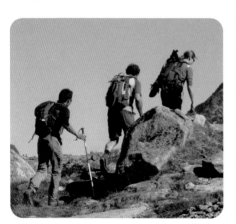

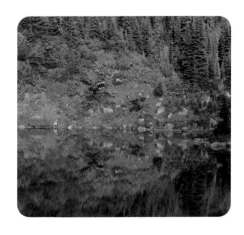

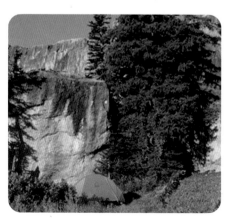

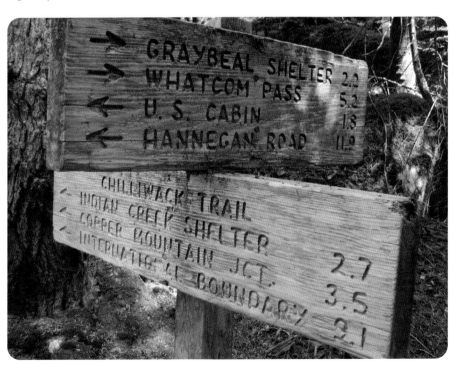

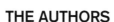

THE AUTHORS

Kathy and Craig are dedicated to each other, and to hiking, in that order. Their second date was a 20-mi (32-km) dayhike in Arizona. Since then they haven't stopped for long.

They've trekked through much of the world's vertical topography, including the Nepalese Himalaya, Patagonian Andes, Spanish Pyrenees, Swiss Alps, Scottish Highlands, Italian Dolomites, and New Zealand Alps. In North America, they've explored the B.C. Coast, Selkirk and Purcell ranges, Montana's Beartooth Wilderness, Wyoming's Grand Tetons, the Colorado Rockies, and the California Sierra.

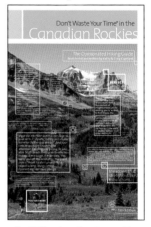

In 1989, they moved from the U.S. to Canada, so they could live near the range that inspired the first of their refreshingly unconventional books: *Don't Waste Your Time in the Canadian Rockies, The Opinionated Hiking Guide*. Its popularity encouraged

them to abandon their careers—Kathy as an ESL teacher, Craig as an ad-agency creative director—and start their own guidebook publishing company: hikingcamping.com.

Kathy and Craig's other books include *Where Locals Hike in the Canadian Rockies*, *Where Locals Hike in the West Kootenay*, *Done In A Day: Whistler*, *Done In A Day: Moab*, *Camp Free in B.C.*, and *Gotta Camp Alberta*.

Partnering with Wilderness Press has empowered Kathy and Craig to explore new publishing horizons, for example the book you now hold in your hands. To create *Hiking from here to Wow: North Cascades*, they hiked more than 2,000 miles (3,220 kms) and ascended elevation equivalent to climbing from sea level to the summit of Mt. Everest nine times. They took more than 1,000 photos and hundreds of pages of field notes.

Other *WOW Guides* by Kathy and Craig will include *Hiking from here to Wow: Utah Canyon Country*. It describes the sensuous landscapes and mysterious archeological sites that most impressed them during their 1,600-mile high-desert odyssey. And it does so in their always refreshing style: honest, literate, entertaining, inspiring.

Though the distances they hike are epic, Kathy and Craig agree that hiking, no matter how far, is the easiest of the many tasks necessary to create a guidebook. What they find most challenging is having to sit at their Canmore, Alberta home, with the Canadian Rockies visible out the window. But they do it every winter, spending twice as much time at their computers—writing, organizing, editing, checking facts—as they do on the trail.

The result is worth it. Kathy and Craig's colorful writing, opinionated commentary, and enthusiasm for the joys of hiking make their guidebooks uniquely helpful and compelling.

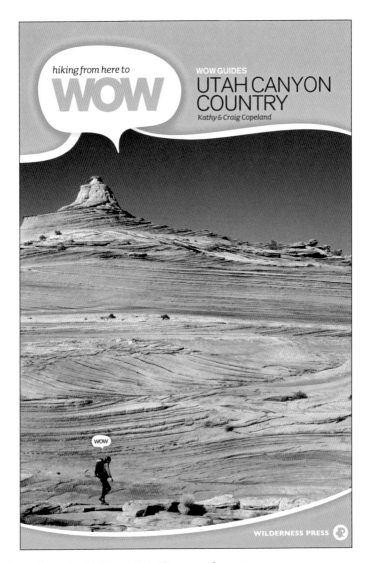

Hiking from here to WOW: Utah Canyon Country
110 Trails to the Wonder Of Wilderness

ISBN: 978-0-89997-452-1   The authors hiked more than 1,600 miles through Zion, Bryce, Escalante-Grand Staircase, Glen Canyon, Grand Gulch, Cedar Mesa, Canyonlands, Moab, Arches, Capitol Reef, and the San Rafael Swell. They took more than 2,000 photos and hundreds of pages of field notes. Then they culled their list of favorite hikes down to 110—each selected for its power to incite awe. Their 480-page book describes where to find the redrock cliffs, slickrock domes, soaring arches, and ancient ruins that make southern Utah unique on planet earth. Like all *WOW Guides*, this one is full-color throughout, with a trail map for each dayhike and backpack trip. First edition, March 2008.

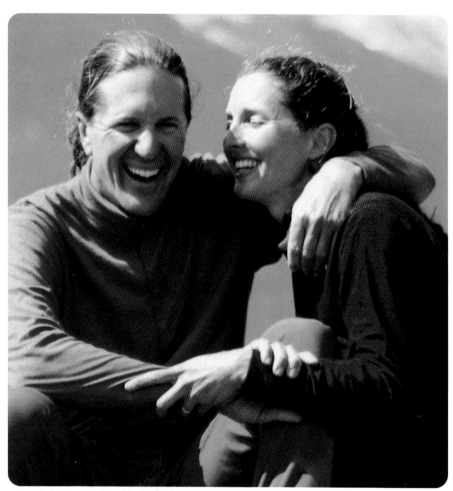

The authors